Contents

About the author

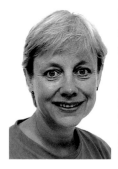

Dr Caroline Bradbeer has been Consultant Genitourinary Physician at Guy's and St Thomas' Hospital, London since 1987. Her research is into thrush, abnormal smears and many aspects of HIV infection. She also works with general practices to improve the sexual health care that they provide.

Introduction

What causes genital symptoms in women?

Women's genital symptoms are often dismissed as having two possible causes: thrush and cystitis. Although these problems are common, they are by no means the only ones to affect this region, and misunderstanding or incorrect treatment can lead to prolonged misery.

For example, antibiotics are usually given to treat a urinary tract infection such as cystitis. If you are actually suffering from a yeast infection (thrush), taking antibiotics may make your symptoms worse by killing the 'friendly' vaginal bacteria that normally keep the yeast infections at bay.

Another example is itching: thrush is the best known cause of itching around the vulva (external female genitals), but other conditions, including skin diseases such as eczema or psoriasis, can also cause it. They require their own different treatments.

Even when the diagnosis is correct and the proper treatment given, it may not be the end of the problem.

Your symptoms may recur and it is often these recurrences that cause the most trouble.

How can this book help?

At some time in your life you will experience symptoms of infection or irritation in the genital area. You may find it a lonely experience because most women do not like to discuss such intimate problems, even with close friends. You might also worry that you could have a sexually transmitted infection.

Trying to find out what the trouble is by examining this part of your body is often difficult, because it is hard for you to see it clearly and it may be embarrassing to ask someone else to look for you. This book is intended to help you if you have genital infections or urinary tract problems so that, where possible, you can work out what is wrong and the best ways to deal with it.

How to use this book

It is difficult to puzzle out what is going on in your body without an understanding of how things work, and how they relate to each other. Most conditions of the female genital tract can easily be understood, and most women can make a fair guess at what is going wrong.

Helping you assess a problem

With a bit of background knowledge, you can often make just as accurate an assessment of the problem as any doctor whom you consult. After all, you know your own body better than a stranger, you have also had longer to think about your symptoms and have more of a vested interest in getting the answer right.

The female sexual organs

This shows a cross-section through the female pelvis. The female sexual organs can be seen together with the position of the bowel and bladder.

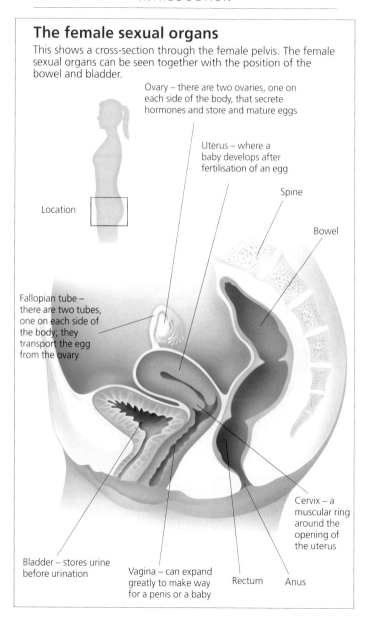

Ovary – there are two ovaries, one on each side of the body, that secrete hormones and store and mature eggs

Uterus – where a baby develops after fertilisation of an egg

Spine

Bowel

Location

Fallopian tube – there are two tubes, one on each side of the body; they transport the egg from the ovary

Cervix – a muscular ring around the opening of the uterus

Bladder – stores urine before urination

Vagina – can expand greatly to make way for a penis or a baby

Rectum

Anus

Understanding what is normal

This book starts with a brief account of the way the female genital region is arranged (what is medically called anatomy) and the way it normally works (physiology). Armed with an understanding of what is normal, it is much easier to work out what is happening when things go wrong.

Common symptoms

The next chapter looks at the symptoms that women commonly notice, what causes them and how to work out the most likely explanation. This chapter is divided into sections, one for each symptom.

Conditions

The conditions themselves are described in detail in the chapter 'Looking for the cause of your symptoms'. Within each section you will also find answers to such questions as: 'Is the diagnosis reliable?', 'What is the treatment?' and 'What are the predisposing factors?'.

Finding out what is wrong

The answers to the above questions explain variations in the accuracy and usefulness of the tests for the condition, tell you what should be done to manage it, and let you know what factors increase your chances of having the condition again.

Seeking help

The final chapters include information on where you should seek help and what to expect, a self-help section, and a glossary to explain unfamiliar or technical terms.

KEY POINTS

■ Women's genital symptoms are often dismissed as having two causes: thrush and cystitis

■ It is important to obtain a correct diagnosis because incorrect treatment can prolong the misery

The female genital region: normal structure and function

The genital region
The vulva
The vulva is the external, visible, outer and inner lips of skin, which partially cover (from front to back) the clitoris, the opening of the urethra (from where urine emerges) and the vaginal opening, called the introitus. Further back still, beyond the vulva, is the anus.

Vulval lubrication
The vulva contains tiny glands that help to keep the skin in this area moist and provide lubrication for sexual intercourse. These glands produce a protective, waterproof film over the skin surface.

If allowed to build up, it can seem as if the vulva has a thick creamy substance over it which could be confused with a vaginal discharge. At other times this waterproofing forms a thin film which can almost be peeled off, especially if the area has been washed with drying agents (astringents) such as some body washes.

How will I know if something is wrong?

Your vulva is a very sensitive piece of skin, with almost as many nerve endings as your lips or mouth, so you will tend to notice immediately when something is wrong.

Most commonly you may notice itching, soreness or pain but, because it is easy to touch the area, you may also detect changes in texture or the development of lumps. Seeing your vulva, however, is not so easy.

You can examine it by crouching over a carefully placed, brightly lit mirror, but this is difficult to arrange even when you are feeling well. As a result, subtle changes are often missed.

Also, because most women seldom examine themselves in this region, they may not know what it normally looks like and so cannot tell whether or not its appearance has changed.

What does it look like?

The normal vulva varies hugely in appearance from woman to woman. The inner and outer lips (labia minora and labia majora) can be anything from hardly present at all to quite large flaps of skin.

The introitus is nearly always surrounded by irregular outgrowths – rather like sea anemone tentacles – which are the remnants of the hymen (the membrane covering the vaginal opening in early life). Even in virgins the hymen is often irregular, and it is a myth that anyone can reliably tell by examining a woman whether or not she is still a virgin.

The vulval area

The vulva is the external visible outer and inner lips of skin. The lips partially conceal the clitoris, the opening of the urethra and the vaginal opening. Your vulva is a very sensitive piece of skin. It has almost as many nerve endings as your lips or mouth, so you will tend to notice immediately when something is wrong.

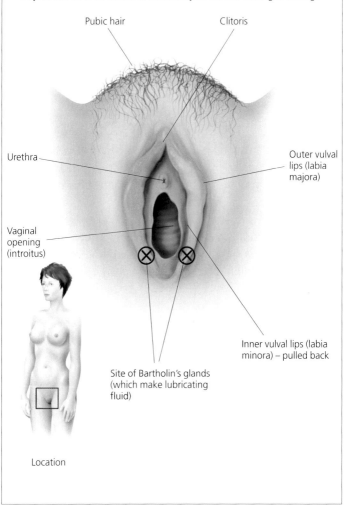

Pubic hair

Clitoris

Urethra

Outer vulval lips (labia majora)

Vaginal opening (introitus)

Inner vulval lips (labia minora) – pulled back

Site of Bartholin's glands (which make lubricating fluid)

Location

The vagina

The vagina is a tube that can lengthen and widen not only to make room for a penis, but also to allow a baby's head and body to go through it. This stretching is possible because of the way the vaginal wall is corrugated, giving it an unusually large surface area.

The vagina contains a complex mix of microbes, proteins, mucus and fluid which make up normal vaginal secretions (see below). This produces an acid, self-cleansing environment which normally keeps a healthy, delicate balance of all its constituents within strict limits.

The vagina opens to the outside world in the middle of the vulva, the introitus. As there are relatively few nerve endings in your vaginal walls, you will not usually feel pain or itching in the vagina itself.

The cervix, uterus, fallopian tubes and ovaries

In general, the deeper inside your body an organ is found, the less sensitive it is to pain and the more difficult it may be for you to pinpoint the exact site of any discomfort. This is true of almost all the organs in your body cavity.

Pain from deep in your pelvis usually feels vague and most people, including their doctors, find it hard to say for certain where it is coming from.

The uterus

Your uterus (womb) is an organ the size and shape of an upside-down pear. It is really a muscle with a central cavity, rather like a very thick-walled bag. It lies deep in your pelvis and connects with the outside via the junction between the cervix (which is Latin for neck) and the vagina.

The fallopian tubes and ovaries

Two fallopian tubes come out of the right and left side of your uterus and the other end of each fallopian tube is loosely in contact with an ovary.

The cervix

Your cervix (neck of the womb) is a muscular ring around the opening of your uterus. It can be likened to a thick rubber band ready to hold the uterus closed around a baby in pregnancy.

The cervix and uterus have very few nerve endings and are not sensitive to ordinary touch. The cervix is not even tender when it is inflamed.

The cervix protrudes into the upper part of the vagina, and the moist membrane lining the uterus and the skin lining the vagina meet on its surface. The uterine lining is thick and red with lots of blood vessels in it (known as columnar epithelium), whereas the vaginal lining is like the skin of the inside of your mouth (squamous epithelium).

The squamocolumnar junction

The actual point where the two types of lining epithelium meet is called the squamocolumnar junction. With changes in hormone levels throughout your reproductive life, it moves its position closer to the cervical canal, or down over the outer cervix.

When the columnar epithelium, which normally lines the uterus, spreads out onto the surface of the cervix, it is known as ectopy or, by its older term, erosion. An ectopy is a fragile area of skin containing lots of secretory glands. The normal fluid and bacteria in the vagina irritate these moist lining cells and cause them to produce increased secretions.

The female reproductive organs

This shows a cross-section through the female reproductive organs. Your uterus or womb is the size and shape of an upside-down pear. It is a muscle with a central cavity connected to the outside by the vagina. It is also connected to the ovaries by two fallopian tubes.

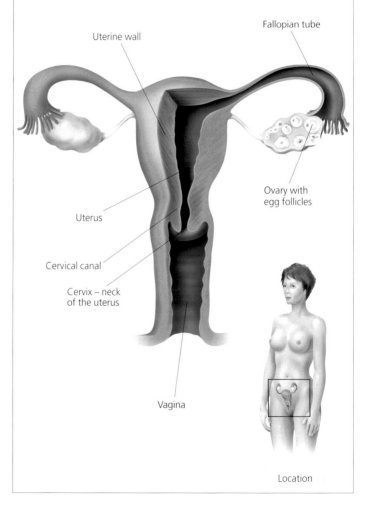

Fallopian tube

Uterine wall

Ovary with egg follicles

Uterus

Cervical canal

Cervix – neck of the uterus

Vagina

Location

It is, however, common to have ectopy and rare for it to be extensive enough to cause troublesome discharge. The exception to this is in pregnancy when oestrogen levels are high and a large ectopy contributes to the increase in secretions at this time.

As the junction between the columnar and squamous cells moves in and out, the skin in the area where the cervix and uterus meet changes type frequently in response to changing hormone levels. A particular area may contain squamous cells on one occasion, but columnar cells on another.

As cancer often develops in places where the cell type fluctuates, this is thought to be why cervical cancer is most likely to develop at the squamocolumnar junction.

The urinary tract
The ureters and bladder
Urine is produced by your kidneys and flows down two muscle-walled tubes known as ureters into your bladder. Your bladder is deep in your pelvis, in front of your uterus and stores urine until you are ready to urinate. It squeezes urine out of your body by contracting its muscular wall.

The urethra
Urine flows out of the bladder through another single tube known, rather confusingly (because of the similarity of the words), as the urethra. The urethra is relatively short in women, but in men it runs the length of the penis and is therefore much longer.

How will I know if something is wrong?
The urethra follows the rule that, the closer a structure is to your body surface, the more sensitive it is.

The kidneys and urinary tract

Your kidneys filter waste products from your blood. This waste is then passed, in solution as urine, into your bladder. Your bladder is located deep in your pelvis in front of your uterus. It stores urine until it is ready for voiding.

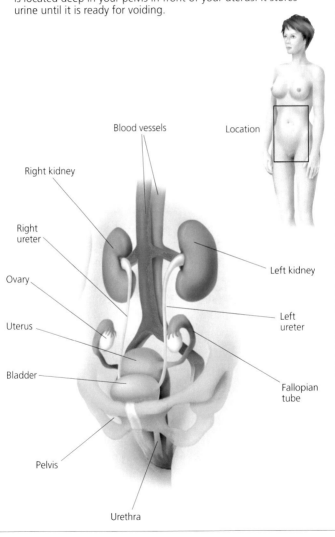

Blood vessels

Location

Right kidney

Right ureter

Left kidney

Ovary

Left ureter

Uterus

Bladder

Fallopian tube

Pelvis

Urethra

The burning pain you feel when urine passes through an inflamed urethra during a urinary tract infection (UTI), commonly called cystitis, is known as dysuria. Inflammation of your bladder, on the other hand, leads to less specific symptoms and you may notice only a dull pelvic or back ache.

The main symptom of a UTI – frequent, painful urination – results from inflammation of your bladder, which then contracts too easily when only a small amount of urine is present.

As urine flows out of your urethra it runs over your vulva. Pain on passing urine is usually attributed to a UTI but, if your vulva itself is sore, urine that is not infected may irritate the tender skin and cause pain as a result of the abrasive chemicals that it contains.

Normal variations in vaginal secretions

The volume and consistency of vaginal secretions are usually under hormonal control. These secretions are most noticeable between puberty and the menopause and are at a maximum during pregnancy.

There is also a smaller increase in the amount of secretions produced each month at the time of ovulation. Sexual excitement will also increase the amount of fluid produced as the vagina lubricates itself ready for intercourse.

Most of the secretions come from the vaginal walls. As a result of its large surface area, the vagina can produce a large volume of fluid.

Some of the normal fluid also comes from the glands around the vulva. The largest of these glands is Bartholin's gland, with one being situated in the rear part of each labium minorum. These glands are important because they can become infected and develop into an abscess.

A small amount of secretion comes from the cervix and uterus.

The range in the amount of normal secretion produced throughout life is vast, but if you are of childbearing age you will probably experience daily staining of your underwear. It is unusual, however, for it to be sufficient to require the regular use of panty liners.

Before puberty

In prepubescent girls, the vagina seems able to resist most of the infections that affect adult women. There are microbes in the vagina but they tend to be different from those in adults and they do not cause problems.

It is rare for a girl to develop genital problems, unless they are caused by skin disease or if the girl's vagina has been subjected to some sort of physical interference or damage.

After puberty

After puberty, a number of healthy bacteria are found in the vagina, of which the most important are lactobacilli. These help keep the vagina acid, compete for available nutrients, and also produce certain chemicals which help to prevent unwanted bacteria and yeasts from becoming established.

Pregnancy

In pregnancy, the cervix, vagina and vulva become larger, with more blood flowing to them and more secretions coming from them. This increase usually starts to become apparent in the first few weeks of pregnancy and may even be the first sign of pregnancy that you notice.

Pregnant women are also more prone to vaginal infections and cystitis because of changes in immunity, and because of the effects of pregnancy hormones.

After the menopause

When oestrogen hormone levels decline at the menopause, the vaginal skin thins, the glands gradually stop working and their secretions decline. As a result, the type of bacteria normally found, including the beneficial lactobacilli, also begins to change.

This leads to dryness, which may be uncomfortable – especially during intercourse – and may make vaginal infections and cystitis more likely.

KEY POINTS

- It is important to be aware of the normal appearance of your genital region so that you can tell more easily whether something is wrong

- Vaginal secretions are normal and vary in appearance and quantity, depending on your age, menstrual cycle and hormone levels

- Your vagina, cervix and uterus do not contain many nerve endings so pain or discomfort originating from within these organs is vague and hard to pinpoint

- Most urinary tract problems cause painful and/or frequent passing of urine

What can go wrong?

Common symptoms and causes

A variety of symptoms can affect the female urinary and lower reproductive tracts. This chapter looks at the symptoms women commonly develop, and their possible causes. Pointers are also given to help you work out the most likely causes.

Vaginal discharge

Women who complain of a vaginal discharge have usually noticed that their normal vaginal secretions have increased, decreased, or changed in colour, consistency or odour. This alteration can be the effect of normal changes in your body, such as in pregnancy, or the result of something going wrong, usually an infection.

Normal (physiological) vaginal fluid

A healthy vagina produces secretions that keep it clean and moist. As the secretions come out at the vulva, they may be called a discharge but, in this context, the term does not imply that there is anything wrong.

The amount of fluid varies as hormone levels change with the menstrual cycle and throughout life. Although it is normal, the change may concern you enough to consult your doctor.

Progesterone-only contraceptive pills (or contraceptive coils containing progesterone – for example, the Mirena intrauterine system) may reduce the amount of physiological secretions and cause concern.

Case history: Jane

Jane, a 14-year-old girl, has just started her periods. At around the same time she notices increased vaginal secretions.

As she and her friends have been made aware, during school lessons and from magazines, that there are infectious causes of vaginal discharge, she worries that she may have something seriously wrong. She tells her mother about her concerns. Jane's mother is able to reassure her that her 'symptom' is perfectly normal now that she has reached puberty.

Case history: Tracy

Tracy is a young woman in her early 20s who has been on the combined oral contraceptive pill for some years. While taking this she has not been ovulating and therefore has not experienced the ovulatory secretion in midcycle for some time.

She decides to stop the pill and after a while notices a vaginal discharge that she interprets as being abnormal. Eventually she makes an appointment to see her doctor who explains that the pill had suppressed her vaginal secretions, which have now returned to normal.

Abnormal vaginal discharge caused by infections

An abnormal vaginal discharge may cause a change in volume or consistency compared with what you have previously experienced. Changes in volume are usually, but not always, an increase above your normal amount. Changes in consistency range from more watery to noticeably thicker.

The most frequent infections that cause abnormal vaginal discharge are caused by *Candida* species (commonly called thrush) or a bacterial imbalance (called bacterial vaginosis or BV). The microbes that cause both of these conditions are present in small amounts in most vaginas and usually cause no symptoms.

When they become problematic, it is sometimes because something (such as recent antibiotic treatment) has upset the normal vaginal balance and allowed one of the microbes to grow more than the others.

Candida
Candida is a yeast (*Candida albicans*) that causes an infection resulting in an inflammatory reaction – swelling and slight oozing of the vaginal walls. This inflammation usually spreads out over the vulva with itching or soreness (see pages 60–73 for more details).

Bacterial vaginosis
Bacterial vaginosis, by contrast, causes little or no inflammation and often no irritation. The main symptom is a discharge and an unpleasant, fishy smell – especially after intercourse (see page 52 for more details).

Trichomonas vaginalis

The third and much rarer infection of the vagina is caused by a single-celled organism (a protozoan) called *Trichomonas vaginalis* (TV). As with the other common infections, it is sometimes symptomless and only detected by chance, for example, on a routine cervical smear.

It usually does cause symptoms, however, and these can be severe enough for the discharge to need a panty liner and cause painful inflammation of the vulva (vulvitis). Unlike the other two common infections (thrush and BV), TV is almost always contracted from a

Vaginal discharge – normal or abnormal?

A healthy vagina produces secretions that keep it clean and moist. The amount of fluid discharged may vary as a result of normal or abnormal causes. This box lists the changes that can increase and decrease normal secretions and the types of infection that can cause an abnormal vaginal discharge.

Normal secretions

Increased	*Decreased*
Puberty	Progesterone contraceptives,
Ovulation	e.g. injections, mini-pill
Pregnancy	Menopause
Sexual arousal	Hysterectomy

Abnormal vaginal discharge

Vaginal infections	*Cervical infections*
Candidiasis	Chlamydial infection
Bacterial vaginosis	Gonorrhoea
Trichomonas vaginalis infection	

sexual partner – it is a sexually transmitted infection (STI) – see pages 73–80 for more details.

Vulval discomfort

Itching is a symptom of mild inflammation and is caused by irritation of nerve endings in the skin. If the irritation increases in severity, it is felt as pain – there is actually a continuum of itching that merges into pain.

It is therefore not always easy to separate the two symptoms. However, specific conditions tend to cause a fairly predictable amount of inflammation and are associated mainly with either itch or soreness.

Vulval itching

Useful clues to the causes of vulval itch are the presence of other symptoms. For example, if you also have an abnormal vaginal discharge, thrush is probably the most likely culprit. If you also have a skin condition, such as eczema, in another part of your body, it may have spread to your vulva.

Some forms of vulval itch can last for months, and have a major effect on your quality of life. Skin conditions such as eczema are a typical example.

Frequently, the problem is a manifestation of the 'itch/scratch cycle'. It begins with an itch. You scratch the area and, after some time, the scratched skin becomes thickened – a common condition known as lichen simplex. This is the body's natural response to rubbing but, unfortunately, thickened skin is itchy.

So the itching and scratching continue. Often, by the time you see a specialist, the original cause of the itch is not apparent or may even have disappeared.

Causes of vulval discomfort

Specific conditions tend to cause a fairly predictable amount of inflammation. Each one is associated mainly with either itch or soreness. The list below groups together those that mainly cause itching and those that mainly cause soreness.

Itching more than soreness
Genital infections
> Candidiasis (thrush)
> Bacterial vaginosis (BV)
> Fungal infections of the groin

Skin conditions
> Eczema
> Psoriasis
> Lichen simplex, as seen in the 'itch/scratch cycle'
> Rare skin conditions, e.g. lichen planus, lichen sclerosus

Soreness more than itching
Genital infections
> *Trichomonas vaginalis* (TV) infection
> Herpes simplex virus infection

Other conditions
> Rare ulcerative diseases, such as Behçet's disease
> Vulvodynia (vulval pain)

Generalised skin conditions

Many women suffering from skin conditions in other parts of their body do not realise that the vulval skin can be affected too. Eczema and psoriasis, for example, commonly affect the vulva and can be difficult to diagnose because they often look and feel different in this area. They may need a specialist dermatologist, and possibly a skin biopsy, to confirm the diagnosis.

Vulval skin conditions

Lichen sclerosus and lichen planus are rare skin conditions affecting the vulva. There is inflammation causing itching for months or years, coupled with increasing discoloration and scarring and shrinkage of the skin of the vulva.

Many women with these conditions experience long and frustrating delays before the diagnosis is made, which is a great shame because the treatment is remarkably simple. The diagnosis is normally made by a biopsy taken by a dermatologist.

The treatment is strong steroid ointment (such as Dermovate) twice daily until the symptoms are under control, followed by occasional applications to keep it at bay. There is a slightly increased risk of the affected skin becoming cancerous and so, because of this and the strong steroids, it needs careful long-term surveillance by experts.

Vulval pain

Generalised pain

Pain in the vulva may be felt over the whole area, especially when it is caused by severe inflammation. The classic cause for generalised pain such as this is the soreness of infection with *Trichomonas vaginalis*. A bad attack of thrush can also be very painful, although you will probably have noticed a worsening itch for several days beforehand.

Vulvodynia is a particularly distressing condition. The word means vulval pain and that really sums up our understanding of it. There is nothing to see – all tests, including biopsies, are normal – but you may feel severe burning.

Interestingly, the condition does seem to respond to a small dose of a drug that interferes with nerve conduction. This drug, amitriptyline, is normally used in much larger doses as an antidepressant because of its action in blocking substances that act as nerve transmitters in the brain.

It is thought, therefore, that vulvodynia may be a disorder of nerve conduction or pain perception, in which the nerves produce a false sensation of pain where there is no obvious cause.

Sores and ulcers

Localised sores on the vulva are commonly the result of herpes simplex infections (see page 80). These vary from small, single ulcers, which are only mildly uncomfortable, to a widespread blistering rash, which is so painful that you can hardly sit or walk. Herpes sores are blisters that break to form small ulcers and they are usually very obvious in appearance.

Other rarer causes of sores or ulcers on the vulva are persistent rubbing, as from a bicycle saddle, or blistering and ulcerating skin conditions (such as Behçet's disease) and some immune-linked conditions (such as Crohn's disease of the intestines) which can also cause genital ulcers.

Pain on passing urine (dysuria)

Pain felt as urine flows through the urethra results from either an irritant effect of urine on the lining of the urethra or unusual sensitivity of the urethral lining.

The most common cause of dysuria is a urinary tract infection (UTI), commonly known as cystitis (see page 38). With a UTI, the urethra is inflamed by the infection, making it sensitive to urine passing through. This discomfort is made worse because the infected urine is more irritant than usual as a result of the infection.

Situations in which urine irritates the urethra without the urethra being inflamed are rare, but can include excessive alcohol in your urine after a drinking binge.

Dysuria also occurs when the urethra or vulva (over which normal urine flows) is inflamed by something other than infection. This may be excessive rubbing and chafing, such as when wearing very tight jeans, or from prolonged sexual intercourse. Inflammation of your vulva can also affect your urethra because these structures are so close together.

Urinary frequency

A different symptom is caused by the irritated muscle in the inflamed bladder wall contracting too readily, so you need to pass urine frequently, and before your

Causes of dysuria

Dysuria (pain on passing urine) is most often caused by one of three main irritants. These are listed below.

- Urine infections
- Sore vulval skin, e.g. infection
- Irritants in the urine

What happens in dysuria

The lining of the urethra can become sensitive. This may be caused by the composition of the urine being overly irritant to the normal urethral lining. It can also be the result of an unusual sensitivity of the urethral lining. Pain is felt as urine flows over the sensitised lining.

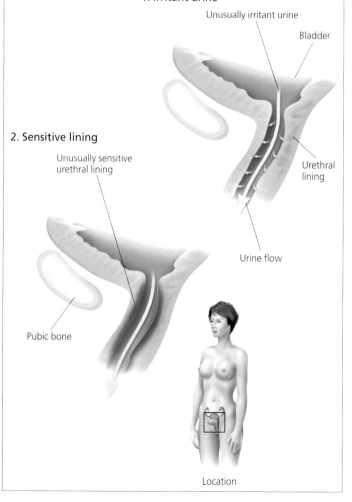

1. Irritant urine

Unusually irritant urine

Bladder

2. Sensitive lining

Unusually sensitive urethral lining

Urethral lining

Urine flow

Pubic bone

Location

bladder is full. This can get so bad that the feeling is almost continuous and, at its extreme, the sensation is so painful and the desire to pass urine so strong that you have to strain to pass only a tiny drop.

This unpleasant condition is still called by an old term, strangury, which is quite descriptive because the bladder seems to squeeze the urine out so strongly that it feels like strangulation. The temptation is to try to avoid this sensation by reducing the volume of your urine still further by not drinking, but this will make the condition worse.

Pelvic pain

Pain felt in your pelvis is usually vague because all your organs are internal and not well supplied with pain receptors. It is therefore difficult to decide where the pain is coming from.

Pelvic pain can originate in your genital, urinary or digestive tract. Probably the best way to sort out vague pelvic pain is to look for other symptoms, which may give a clue to its origin.

For example, an abnormal vaginal discharge or irregular periods might point to your uterus and fallopian tubes as a likely source. Urinary symptoms would suggest your bladder, and diarrhoea or constipation your bowel.

Irritable bowel syndrome, when the pain comes from the lower bowel, is a very common cause of pelvic pain in young women. It should always be considered when the pain is long lasting, especially if there are bowel symptoms (see the Family Doctor Book *Understanding Irritable Bowel Syndrome*).

Organs involved in pelvic pain

Pelvic pain can originate in your genital, urinary or digestive tract. The most likely sources of the pain are listed below.

- Uterus
- Fallopian tubes and ovaries
- Bladder
- Rectum and large bowel

Pain in your uterus, fallopian tubes and ovaries

Pain in the pelvis is frequently caused by a problem with your uterus, fallopian tubes or ovaries (your upper genital tract). You will not feel any pain if your cervix or upper vagina (rather than vulva) is inflamed.

A very inflamed cervix will exude mucus and pus but, as it is such a small structure, it produces only a small amount. This discharge then mixes with your normal vaginal secretions, and even if you have a very inflamed cervix it may go unnoticed, unless complications set in.

Upper genital tract pain is often described as similar to period cramps or early labour. If your uterus and fallopian tubes are tender, this can be detected during an internal examination by rocking your cervix to and fro (and hence your uterus) which will cause discomfort.

Movement of your cervix in this way also occurs in vaginal intercourse, so if you feel deep pain during intercourse you may have a problem in your upper genital tract. The box on page 31 lists the possible causes of upper genital tract pain.

Possible origin of pelvic pain

Pain from the internal organs is usually dull and focused on the midline of the abdomen. The origin is usually hard to determine because the organs are concealed in the abdomen and they are not well supplied with pain sensors. Probably the best way to sort out where your pain is coming from is to look at the nature of your other symptoms.

Pain from the internal organs of the abdomen is usually dull and focused on the midline of the abdomen.

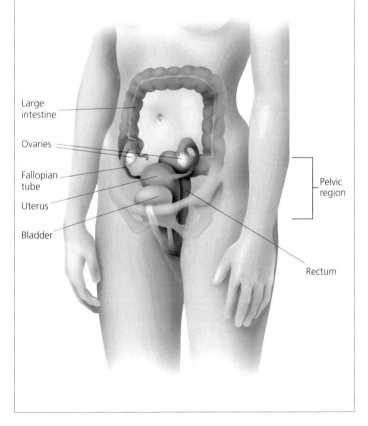

Large intestine

Ovaries

Fallopian tube

Uterus

Bladder

Pelvic region

Rectum

Causes of upper genital tract pain

The upper genital tract comprises the uterus, fallopian tubes and ovaries. Upper genital tract pain is often described as like a menstrual cramp or early labour. Its causes can include:

Physiological pain
- Midcycle (ovulation pain)
- Period pain
- Early pregnancy

Pelvic inflammatory disease (PID)
- Chlamydial infection (see page 101)
- Gonorrhoea (see page 101)
- Other infections

Endometriosis (see page 109)

Bleeding or twisting of:
- Fibroids
- Ovarian cysts (see page 111)

Sexual problems

Sexual problems can have physical or psychological causes. The medical word for painful intercourse is dyspareunia.

This is divided into superficial dyspareunia (pain on penetration felt at the entrance to the vagina) and deep dyspareunia (pain during sexual intercourse felt deep in the pelvis). Deep dyspareunia is likely to have a physical cause, whereas superficial dyspareunia is more likely to have a psychological or sexual cause.

There is a chicken-and-egg quality to many sexual problems and frequently also a vicious cycle (see Case history below). A common scenario is that you may not become sexually excited because you are sore or have thrush, and will therefore not become adequately lubricated.

If intercourse still takes place, there will be physical friction, making you more uncomfortable and sore. The discomfort will put you off the idea of intercourse, so you are even less likely to become adequately lubricated next time and it will be even more uncomfortable.

It may have started with a physical reason for soreness but it ends with a psychological one caused by tension. On the other hand, you may have been tense to start with but assumed the pain was the result of an attack of thrush or a bladder infection.

Recurrent genital problems can therefore cause sexual problems, but, in addition, sexual problems can appear to have a physical cause. In either of these situations it may at first appear, to both you and your doctor, that the problem is wholly physical. Psychosexual counsellors recognise this phenomenon and often have to work hard to unravel it.

Case history: Simone

Simone (age 33) had recently been sexually assaulted. She was worried about the prospect of resuming sexual intercourse with her regular partner. When they tried, she was so tense that penetration was difficult and painful.

However, she and her partner continued despite the pain that she was feeling. As intercourse was painful, her subconscious worked harder to prevent it happening by making her tense up her muscles even further; she became even more upset and penetration became more painful.

Possible origin of painful intercourse

The medical word for painful intercourse is dypareunia. This is divided into superficial dypareunia (pain on penetration felt at the entrance to the vagina) and deep dypareunia (pain during sexual intercourse felt deep in the pelvis).

1. Superficial dyspareunia

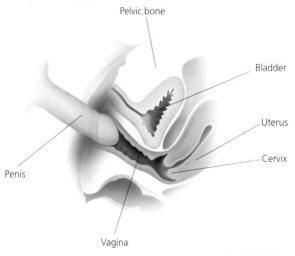

Pelvic bone

Bladder

Uterus

Cervix

Penis

Vagina

2. Deep dyspareunia

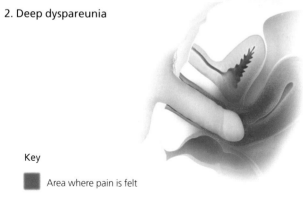

Key

Area where pain is felt

The next time her partner suggested intercourse she tensed up even before they started. She did not want intercourse, she was not lubricated, and she became so tense that her inner thigh and pelvic muscles went into spasm, and he was unable to penetrate at all.

This condition is known as vaginismus. Simone told her doctor that she had a sore vulva, but after discussion they were able to establish that the soreness was a result of her tension and not the other way round.

Problems before puberty

Young girls with an itchy vulva may have itchy skin conditions or fungal sweat rashes. It is uncommon for a girl to develop a vaginal discharge before the onset of puberty.

If she does, a common cause is a foreign body in her vagina, such as a marble or some other small object that she has introduced herself. Other causes are related to poor hygiene, when more than the normal numbers of bowel organisms take over the vagina.

Vaginal discharge in girls raises the possibility, however unlikely, of sexual abuse. In this context, a discharge could be the result of a sexually transmitted infection (STI), such as gonorrhoea.

Gonorrhoea in girls affects the vaginal walls, unlike in grown women (where it infects the cervix) and can therefore cause a vaginal discharge. Gonorrhoea in girls is very rare, however.

Genital examination of young girls is an undesirable and traumatic procedure, not just for the girl but also for her parents and even for the doctor. It may, however, be necessary to determine the reason for a vaginal discharge. If this distressing procedure is necessary it can be carried out under general anaesthetic.

Any situation like this involving a child will need the health professional to work to the Child Protection Regulations and this may involve getting a specialist in child health to see the girl.

Problems during pregnancy

Pregnant women have an increased chance of developing candidal infection, as a result of their increased oestrogen levels, but this has no effect on the outcome of their pregnancy.

Bacterial vaginosis, by contrast, has been increasingly linked to premature labour, and even to miscarriage. The evidence for these links in pregnancy is still not entirely clear.

However, many doctors currently recommend that if you have BV when you are pregnant you should be treated for it. At other times, BV is no more than a nuisance.

Gonorrhoea and chlamydial infection may also be related to premature labour, but the main concern is after delivery. Both infections can spread to the pelvic organs after labour, causing pelvic inflammatory disease (PID) (see page 105).

Will the baby be affected?

The baby can be infected while passing down the birth canal and picks up the mother's infection to develop conjunctivitis (sticky eye). Rarely, babies can develop chlamydial pneumonia and, even more rarely, baby girls can develop a vaginal gonorrhoeal infection.

Genital warts can also be transmitted to babies at delivery. In this case the child's mother usually has, or has had, warts. Occasionally, a girl baby or toddler develops warts on her vulva.

As genital warts are sexually transmissible, these may raise questions about sexual abuse. However, in the vast majority of cases the warts have come from the mother, usually from contact with the mother's genitals during birth.

Problems after the menopause

Normal vaginal secretions decrease after the menopause, unless you are on hormone replacement therapy (HRT). The dryness can be quite marked and a dry vulva and vagina often become sore, making sex uncomfortable.

At the menopause you go through changes that are both physical and psychological, and this experience may alter the way that you perceive your genitals. You may regard pain during intercourse or genital discomfort as part of the menopause package, and these symptoms then reinforce any negative feelings that you may have about yourself.

You may find that you have entered into the vicious cycle of dry intercourse, making you less interested in sex, so you are less easily aroused and drier the next time that you attempt it. As a result, you may begin to avoid sex altogether. Simple measures such as lubricants often help. Oestrogen creams, for insertion into the vagina, are available on prescription and can relieve dryness.

HRT is usually prescribed for a short time around the menopause for its beneficial effects on menopausal symptoms such as hot flushes and night sweats. HRT also has an effect on the vagina so that it becomes moister and returns more closely to its premenopausal state (see *Understanding the Menopause and HRT*, another book in the Family Doctor series).

KEY POINTS

- Pain on passing urine is usually caused by a urinary tract infection

- Your vulva is highly sensitive and any itching or soreness in this area can cause much distress

- It is normal to have vaginal secretions; it is a concern only if the discharge is excessive, greatly reduced or has an offensive smell

- Pelvic pain is often vague and hard to pinpoint

- Sexual problems and physical genital problems can easily be confused

- Girls and women are susceptible to different urinary and genital problems at various life stages

- Genital infections in pregnancy may cause premature labour or be passed on to your newborn baby

- The lowered hormone levels that occur after the menopause reduce normal vaginal secretions, causing discomfort and dryness; HRT can, to a certain extent, reverse this pattern

Looking for the cause of your symptoms

Urinary tract infections
What are they?
The term 'urinary tract infections' (UTIs) and the word 'cystitis' are often used to mean the same thing. Strictly speaking, however, cystitis just means an inflammation of the bladder (which may be the result of infection or irritation), whereas UTI implies that any or all parts of the urinary tract are infected. UTI is therefore probably the better term.

UTIs are common in women from puberty onwards. One in five women experiences a UTI at some time in her life.

Normal urine is said to be 'sterile' because it does not contain bacteria, although it may contain viruses, which do not cause UTIs. The most common bacteria to infect urine are those that normally live harmlessly in your bowel or on the skin of your vulva.

Urinary tract infection

Any part or all of the urinary tract can be infected and this is called a urinary tract infection (UTI). It is sometimes called cystitis but that is strictly inflammation of just the bladder. Several types of bacteria are commonly responsible for the infection. In about 75 per cent of cases the cause is the bacterium *Escherichia coli*, which originates in the bowel.

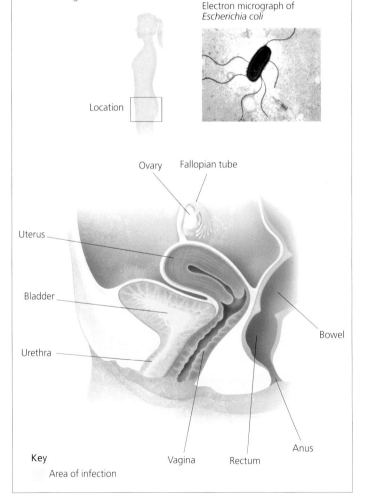

Electron micrograph of
Escherichia coli

Location

Ovary   Fallopian tube

Uterus

Bladder

Urethra

Bowel

Key

Area of infection

Vagina   Rectum   Anus

Although UTIs are not sexually transmitted, they are more common if you are sexually active because intercourse may push bacteria up into your urethra – a woman's urethra is relatively short – and from there to your bladder.

Although several different types of bacteria are commonly responsible for UTIs, 75 per cent of cases are caused by a type of *Escherichia coli* that originates in the bowel, where it is harmless. This should not be confused with the type of *E. coli* that is occasionally responsible for outbreaks of food poisoning.

How are UTIs diagnosed?

The diagnosis of a UTI depends on finding a significant number (usually more than 10,000 bacteria per millilitre of urine) of a particular bacterium (see box on page 43) in your urine. To do this, urine has to be cultured in a laboratory to see what organisms grow. This takes time so it is often better to start treatment as soon as possible.

A UTI can be diagnosed on the basis of symptoms alone, backed up by simple 'on-the-spot' urine tests. These tests are readily available in your GP's surgery, and family planning and genitourinary medicine (GUM) clinics.

'On-the-spot' tests

'On-the-spot' tests can detect chemical changes in your urine that result when bacteria multiply in your bladder. For example, bacteria in the urine break down the natural urine waste product, urea, to form the chemicals, nitrites.

Bacteria also attract white blood cells into the area to fight the infection. When these die they release the

Diagnosis by culturing a swab in a laboratory

To prove the diagnosis the urine has to be cultured to see which organisms will grow. This takes time and the techniques are available only in a microbiology lab. The illustrations below outline the procedure.

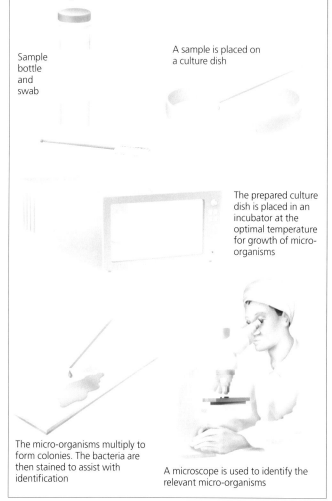

Sample bottle and swab

A sample is placed on a culture dish

The prepared culture dish is placed in an incubator at the optimal temperature for growth of micro-organisms

The micro-organisms multiply to form colonies. The bacteria are then stained to assist with identification

A microscope is used to identify the relevant micro-organisms

enzyme leucocyte esterase. Bacterial infection also produces inflammation of the bladder walls, which then ooze small amounts of protein and red blood cells.

Dipstick tests

The simplest 'on-the-spot' tests for UTIs are special reagent dipsticks that have a series of absorbent pads impregnated with detector chemicals. The stick is dipped into your urine and colour changes are compared with a chart to read the result.

These dipsticks can detect one or more of the following signs of an active infection:

- Nitrites from urea breakdown

- Leucocyte esterase from white blood cells

- Protein and blood from inflammation.

The advantage of these urinary dipstick tests is that they give immediate results. They cannot, however, definitely confirm that an infection is present and they cannot tell which bacterium is involved or which particular antibiotic will kill it.

Is the diagnosis reliable?

Confirmation of the guilty bacterium is not always easy. The specimen of urine has to be fresh and kept in a fridge to prevent other skin bacteria from multiplying in it and confusing the results.

Also the bacteria must be kept alive until they reach the laboratory. If a specimen is taken – for example, on a hot Friday afternoon – and left in a fridge over the weekend, two things may happen to affect the true result:

Bacteria that cause urinary tract infections (UTIs)

Many different bacteria can cause a UTI. The diagnosis of a UTI is confirmed by a laboratory test finding significant (usually about 10,000 or more bacteria per millilitre of urine) numbers of a bacterium in the urine. Possible bacteria include:

- *Escherichia coli*
- *Proteus* species
- *Pseudomonas* species
- *Staphylococcus epidermidis*
- *Klebsiella* species
- *Streptococcus* species

1 First, the bacteria may die, so that none are detected by the time the specimen reaches the laboratory.
2 Second, if other bacteria get into the specimen, even in small numbers, they may multiply over the weekend, in which case these innocent bacteria will be detected when the test is done.

False-negative results
Sometimes your symptoms seem typical of a UTI, and resolve with antibiotic treatment, but laboratory tests do not show that your urine was infected. An explanation for this may be that insufficient bacteria survived to meet the significant number needed to confirm an infection in the laboratory.

Inadequate flushing of the urinary tract

This shows a bladder with a normal flow of urine and one with inadequate flushing. Infections do not usually take hold in the urinary tract because bacteria are constantly flushed away by the flow of urine. The immune system is generally able to cope with the few bacteria that do creep in.

Inadequate flushing

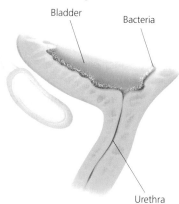

Bladder

Bacteria

Urethra

Inadequate flushing of the urinary tract allows bacteria to colonise and cause symptoms

Normal flushing

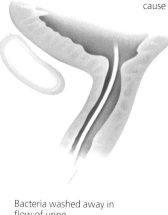

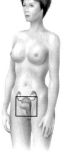

Bacteria washed away in flow of urine

Location

Bacteria that cause urinary tract infections (UTIs)

Many different bacteria can cause a UTI. The diagnosis of a UTI is confirmed by a laboratory test finding significant (usually about 10,000 or more bacteria per millilitre of urine) numbers of a bacterium in the urine. Possible bacteria include:

- *Escherichia coli*
- *Proteus* species
- *Pseudomonas* species
- *Staphylococcus epidermidis*
- *Klebsiella* species
- *Streptococcus* species

1 First, the bacteria may die, so that none are detected by the time the specimen reaches the laboratory.
2 Second, if other bacteria get into the specimen, even in small numbers, they may multiply over the weekend, in which case these innocent bacteria will be detected when the test is done.

False-negative results

Sometimes your symptoms seem typical of a UTI, and resolve with antibiotic treatment, but laboratory tests do not show that your urine was infected. An explanation for this may be that insufficient bacteria survived to meet the significant number needed to confirm an infection in the laboratory.

Urine samples almost always contain some bacteria from your vulva. When a laboratory detects a small number of bacteria, especially if there is a mixture of types, they may discount the finding and report the urine as containing 'contaminants only'.

This is because they assumed that the bacteria multiplied in (or contaminated) the sample after it was taken. This practice reduces the number of tests that appear to be positive (false positives) when they are not, for example, because of contamination. The downside of this is that the tests may report a few genuine UTIs as negative (false negatives).

Ironically, if a woman suspects that she has a UTI and drinks a lot of fluid to help flush out the infection, she may also dilute the bacteria and get a false-negative result. A helpful deciding factor in this case would be the presence of dead white blood cells. If enough of these are seen in the urine under the laboratory microscope they indicate that a true infection was likely.

Confusion with other disorders or contamination

The symptoms of a UTI, dysuria (pain on passing urine), pelvic discomfort or urinary frequency (passing urine more frequently than usual), are also symptoms of many other urinary and genital disorders. These may be incorrectly diagnosed as a UTI.

'On-the-spot' urine tests can also be misleading. For example, there may be other reasons for finding protein or red blood cells in the urine, such as when the sample is contaminated with menstrual blood or vaginal discharge.

What makes you more likely to have UTIs?

Infections do not generally take hold in your urinary tract because bacteria are constantly flushed away by the flow of urine. Your immune system can usually cope with the few bacteria that do creep in.

Bacteria are more likely to become established and multiply in your urinary tract under certain conditions. These are when you have a reduced urine flow (as in dehydration or kidney failure), incomplete emptying of your bladder or reduced immunity. Examples of when there is reduced immunity are pregnancy, diabetes, steroid therapy and HIV infection.

Incomplete bladder emptying can be caused by pressure from the outside, deforming the bladder wall. This can happen when a pregnant uterus presses on the bladder or when abnormalities or weaknesses of the bladder wall (or, higher up, of the ureter or kidney) prevent complete emptying.

These abnormalities are often the result of childbirth or they may be congenital (present from birth. Damage after an accident, multiple sclerosis or surgery can also interfere with proper bladder emptying by interrupting the nerve supply, which would normally coordinate the time at which and the way in which your bladder contracts.

Other abnormalities that prevent complete flushing of the system are bladder stones and wart-like growths on the bladder wall (papillomas), which harbour bacteria in their crevices. Papillomas can also bleed slightly and must be monitored because they can develop into cancer.

Inadequate flushing of the urinary tract

This shows a bladder with a normal flow of urine and one with inadequate flushing. Infections do not usually take hold in the urinary tract because bacteria are constantly flushed away by the flow of urine. The immune system is generally able to cope with the few bacteria that do creep in.

Inadequate flushing

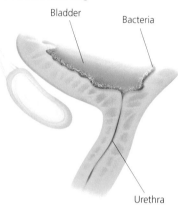

Bladder

Bacteria

Urethra

Inadequate flushing of the urinary tract allows bacteria to colonise and cause symptoms

Normal flushing

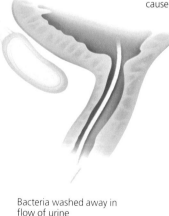

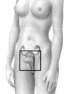

Bacteria washed away in flow of urine

Location

Factors that increase the risk of UTIs

Your urinary tract is flushed regularly by the flow of urine. Any bacteria that may get in are usually dealt with by your immune system. You are more susceptible to a UTI in any of the situations listed below.

Inadequate 'flushing' of the urinary tract
- Poor urine flow, as in dehydration or kidney failure
- Anatomical abnormalities: congenital (present from birth, such as horseshoe-shaped kidney) acquired (e.g. after surgery)
- Poor bladder emptying, as in old age or multiple sclerosis

Reduced resistance to bacteria
- Pregnancy
- Reduced immunity, as in HIV infection
- Other illnesses, e.g. diabetes

Bacteria able to 'hide' in the bladder
- Urinary stones
- Bladder papillomas (wart-like growths)
- Foreign bodies, such as urinary catheters

What is the treatment?

If you have a UTI you may be prescribed an antibiotic before the test results are available. It may later turn out that the bacterium was resistant to the chosen antibiotic, but at the start of treatment you have to rely on the doctor's 'best guess' as to which antibiotic will work.

Antibiotics

Several different classes of antibiotic are available. Some work by killing bacteria (for example, by puncturing their cell walls) and others work by stopping bacteria from multiplying so the body's immune system can overpower them.

An uncomplicated UTI should get better with a very short course of antibiotics – two days at most. If it doesn't, the possibilities are a wrong diagnosis, a complication or the bacteria being resistant to the chosen antibiotic.

Sometimes, surprisingly, bacteria are still destroyed by an antibiotic to which laboratory tests suggest it is resistant. This may be because large doses of an antibiotic can sometimes overcome the bacterium's resistance and kill it anyway.

Drinking

It is important not just to rely on the antibiotic, but also to make sure that you increase your urine production to flush out the bacteria. You should increase your fluid intake and empty your bladder frequently. By drinking more water, your urine will be weaker and less irritant.

Discomfort and burning can also be reduced by making your urine more alkaline. Several commercial powders are available to reduce the acidity of urine, e.g. Cymalon.

Drinking cranberry juice has been recommended for both the treatment and prevention of UTIs. A substance in the husk of the berries is thought to be the helpful agent. It interferes with *E. coli* sticking to the urethral and bladder walls, thus helping urine to wash it out.

Even if the bacterium in your urine is not *E. coli*, cranberry juice is a palatable form in which to take the necessary volume of fluid. It may well be effective and it does no harm.

Are there any complications?

A bad infection of your bladder can spread up one or other of your ureters into a kidney, causing a severe kidney infection known as pyelonephritis. This is especially likely to happen if:

- your ureter is dilated (more open – as naturally occurs in pregnancy)

- the urine flow down your ureter is slow

- you have some anatomical abnormality (such as an extra ureter), which encourages pooling of infected urine.

What about your sexual partner?

UTIs are not passed on sexually and there is no need for your sexual partner to worry. The only sexual link is that UTIs occur more frequently after intercourse. This is because bacteria are pushed into your bladder as a result of sex.

What about recurrent UTIs?

Repeated infections, or recurrences, may be related to one or other of the abnormalities mentioned above. If you have recurrent UTIs you should have tests for these abnormalities.

These include careful urine testing and ultrasound (or an X-ray) of the urinary tract. Often, however, nothing abnormal is found.

How can I stop it recurring?

Prevention of recurrences is difficult, but there are many strategies to choose from, depending on your circumstances. The most obvious one is to increase your fluid intake to at least two litres spread over each day.

You may also find that emptying your bladder immediately after sexual intercourse prevents UTIs. Many women find 'double micturition' is helpful – this involves emptying your bladder, then standing up and walking about for a few moments, and then trying to empty your bladder again.

Other general advice includes wiping your anal area away from your urethra (backwards), after opening your bowels. You should also avoid douching (squirting fluid into your vagina).

If UTIs are frequent, antibiotics can be taken whenever there is a precipitating factor, such as sexual intercourse. Sometimes antibiotics need to be taken daily to prevent very frequent recurrences.

The urethral syndrome

This is found mainly in women and is a poorly understood condition. If you suffer from the urethral syndrome, you will have all the symptoms of a UTI but, when your urine is tested in the laboratory, nothing abnormal is found.

The condition may have a variety of causes:

- A true infection may be present but with too few bacteria for the laboratory to confirm an infection.

- The irritation may be confined to your urethra, perhaps as a result of an infection that has not spread as far as your bladder. In this case, the infection often seems to be brought on by rubbing from clothing or by sexual intercourse.

- There may be no infection and the symptoms result entirely from increased sensitivity of the urethra, either from rubbing or from an unknown cause.

Whatever the cause, it is more common in sexually active women.

You may find that changing your position for sexual intercourse, so that you are on top, or using extra lubricant, such as KY Jelly, is helpful. Other general measures described above for dealing with recurrent UTIs, such as careful attention to the timing and thoroughness of bladder emptying, can also help.

Chemical cystitis

Although an inflamed bladder is commonly caused by a UTI, there are other causes of cystitis without infection. The two most common of these are related to cancer therapy.

Chemotherapy drugs for cancer are designed to stop cells dividing. They tend to be very irritant and many of them are passed out in the urine, where they can inflame the bladder to cause so-called 'chemical cystitis'.

The other common cancer treatment is radiotherapy, in which powerful X-rays are directed at the cancer to kill the cells. Any normal cells in the same area can also become damaged, so radiotherapy to the pelvis – for example, to treat cancer of the cervix – can also inflame the bladder wall, causing a very severe form of cystitis.

Bacterial vaginosis
What is it?

Bacterial vaginosis (BV) is responsible for the most common type of abnormal vaginal discharge. It is caused by the overgrowth of a mixture of bacteria that are often normally present in small quantities.

When you have BV, the normal bacteria multiply and replace many of the other natural organisms found in the vagina. There is very little inflammation, and itching and soreness are not a major feature. You may have mild irritation from the watery vaginal discharge that is usually present.

Attacks of BV will go away in time in most people. At other times attacks may never become the full-blown condition.

Typical smell

Some of the bacteria live anaerobically (without the need for oxygen) which means that they have an unusual metabolism and break down proteins to chemicals known as amines. This makes your normally acid vaginal secretions more alkaline, and it releases an ammonia-like smell resembling rotting fish.

The fishy smell is worse when the discharge is mixed with alkaline secretions such as urine or semen. You may therefore notice the smell most after unprotected vaginal intercourse or when passing urine. You may even think it is your urine that smells.

There is a male, locker-room myth that it is normal for women to smell fishy. Some women also believe that a fishy odour is normal and this means that a woman with BV may not recognise that anything is wrong.

Bacterial vaginosis

Bacterial vaginosis (BV) is responsible for the most common type of abnormal vaginal discharge. It is caused by the overgrowth of a mixture of bacteria, including *Gardnerella vaginalis*, that are often normally present in small quantities. When you have BV, however, these bacteria multiply and replace many of the other natural organisms found in the vagina. The yellow area shows the infected vagina.

Electron micrograph of *Gardnerella vaginalis*

Location

Bladder

Uterus

Pubic bone

Urethra

Vagina

Rectum

Anus

Key

Area of infection

Care in pregnancy

Bacterial vaginosis is not harmful except in pregnancy. Researchers have found a link between BV and premature labour and pre-term birth. There is also a suggested link, less convincing as yet, between BV and miscarriage.

However, no one is sure whether this link is because BV causes premature labour or whether there is some other common factor. Even so, many doctors now play safe and prescribe antibiotics to pregnant women with BV.

How is it diagnosed?

There are several ways to confirm a diagnosis of BV, some of which can be done on the spot, for example, the typical change in the acidity (pH) of the vagina can be confirmed by testing a sample of discharge with ordinary laboratory litmus paper.

Another simple test is to mix a sample of your discharge with an alkaline substance such as sodium hydroxide (caustic soda). This releases the typical fishy, amine odour, and forms the basis for the 'sniff test' and other commercially available tests.

Studying a stained slide of secretions under the microscope is the best way to diagnose BV. This test is frequently carried out in specialist, genitourinary medicine clinics, but it requires expertise and a microscope, which are not available in other settings.

The advantage is that the microscopy can detect grades of BV. There are two main ways to classify BV changes in the discharge; the most used one is the Hay–Ison classification which gives three stages from 0 to 3, where 3 is full-blown BV.

If you have grade 2, you may still notice some changes and often have a smell. Sometimes this will get better by itself; at other times it progresses to grade 3.

In a GP's practice the usual test for BV is done on a sample sent to the laboratory for testing. The results of this will take at least 48 hours to come back. Your GP will either wait for these or make a diagnosis and give you treatment on the basis of your symptoms and his or her examination findings.

Is the diagnosis reliable?

The microbiological swab test for BV searches for a bacterium called *Gardnerella vaginalis*. Although this bacterium is almost always present in BV, it is not present in 100 per cent of cases.

If *Gardnerella vaginalis* is present, it is a useful pointer to the diagnosis but does not prove that the condition is BV. Equally, its absence does not exclude the possibility of BV.

Diagnosis of BV is not easy when the pH test, the sniff test and the slide test do not all agree. Some may point to a diagnosis of BV and others away from it.

Diagnostic uncertainty is also not helped by the fact that BV is so common that some women accept it as a normal state. Others with no sign of BV become convinced that they have an odour and that everyone around them can smell it.

It seems that these women have an oversensitive sense of smell for BV. Sometimes it is a sign of psychological problems where an obsession that they smell is due to troubles in their relationship or even self-loathing.

Case history: Margaret
Margaret, age 35, an accountant, had been diagnosed

several times with BV in the past and had become obsessive about her odour. All the tests were negative and the examining doctor and nurse could smell nothing. She was unconvinced and was only helped by repeated negative tests, a second opinion and a long discussion with a counsellor.

Case history: Angela

A 23-year-old hairdresser, Angela, with no symptoms had a routine screening for sexually transmitted infections (STIs). She was found to have BV and her doctor prescribed some treatment. When Angela returned to her doctor for a follow-up appointment, she reported that she noticed no difference but her boyfriend had told her 'The smell's gone'.

What makes you more likely to suffer from BV?

It is not clear what triggers an attack of BV. The foreign body effect seems to be a factor – that is, when there is a 'foreign' bit of material (such as a forgotten tampon), or even a severe inflammatory disease process, that upsets the normal balance of microbes (the flora) in the vagina.

A forgotten tampon is very effective at changing the flora in the vagina. It causes a foul smell that has elements of the odour of BV but is far more putrid. Thankfully, however, bacterial imbalances normalise once the offending tampon has been removed.

Infection with *Trichomonas vaginalis* (TV) often occurs with BV. As TV is the more serious of the two and the treatment is the same for both, this is dealt with later (see page 77).

If you have severe attacks of genital herpes (see page 80), you will also often have BV. It will disappear when the herpes attack resolves.

Until recently, the contraceptive coil (intrauterine contraceptive device – IUCD) was linked to BV. The latest studies do not confirm this link, although there is a suggestion that, if a woman with an IUCD changes her sexual partner, she may be more likely than a woman without an IUCD to develop BV. The explanation for this finding is still unclear.

Many feminine hygiene practices have been accused of causing, or encouraging, the development of BV. Many of them are also said to do the same for thrush (see page 60). The following have all been blamed:

- using soap on your genital area (especially strongly scented varieties)

- using bath additives

- douching your vagina (squirting fluid into your vagina)

- using vaginal deodorants.

These substances are thought to upset the normal self-cleansing mechanism of your vagina. Also, by disturbing the acid balance of your vaginal flora, they can cause overgrowth of the organisms that cause BV.

Unfortunately, in many cases, none of these factors is present and there is no explanation for the BV.

What is the treatment?

The object of treatment is to return your vaginal flora to normal. This is done by killing the abnormal, anaerobic bacteria, to leave room in the vagina for the normal ones (normal flora) to grow back.

Metronidazole

The usual treatment is metronidazole, an antibiotic that works almost exclusively against anaerobes without affecting the healthy, desirable vaginal flora – or even other problematic bacteria such as those normally causing UTIs. Metronidazole is therefore described as a 'narrow-spectrum antibiotic' and can be given as tablets or as a vaginal gel.

The side effects of metronidazole are nausea and an unpleasant reaction with alcohol. (There is a popular belief that you should avoid alcohol with all antibiotics but this is not so – metronidazole is about the only antibiotic that requires you to avoid alcohol, and even with metronidazole there is only about a 10% chance that you will be ill if you drink while taking it.) However, the side effects are minimised further if you use the drug in a gel formulation directly into your vagina.

Clindamycin

A broader-spectrum antibiotic (one that kills a wider range of different bacteria), clindamycin, is available in cream form for insertion into the vagina (Dalacin Cream). It is just as effective as oral antibiotics in eradicating BV.

How is the antibiotic chosen?

The choice usually depends on whether you prefer to take drugs by mouth or insert them, and of course on their price and availability. Both metronidazole and clindamycin are given as five- or seven-day courses and metronidazole can be given in a single large dose of two grams.

Am I likely to have another genital infection?

Some people believe that, if you have BV, you are also more likely to have other genital infections. There is not much evidence to back this up. However, if you suspect that you are at risk, it is worth you and your partner being tested, because some STIs, such as chlamydial infection, are hard to detect in women.

What about your sexual partner?

Bacterial vaginosis is more common in sexually active women, especially, some research suggests, in lesbian women. However, it is not passed on sexually between partners and treating her male sexual partner for BV has no effect on a woman's disease.

What about recurrent BV infection?

Bacterial vaginosis often comes back (a recurrent attack). The usual story is that each time you have an attack it gets better with therapy, but then returns weeks or months later, often time after time. As there is rarely an obvious reason for this, preventing attacks can be difficult.

You should, of course, try to get rid of any of the predisposing causes, outlined above, and to be careful with other practices, such as washing, to see if that helps. If you are still getting recurrences after the known triggers have been removed, there is little more that can be done.

There are two courses of action. You can put up with the symptoms until they go of their own accord, which they will in time. Alternatively, you could make an arrangement with your GP to have a prescription for your preferred medication whenever you recognise a return of the symptoms.

I usually arrange for women with recurrent BV to have a couple of doses of BV treatment to keep at home so they can treat themselves as soon as possible. BV is, after all, not really an illness and it is important for the sufferer to feel that she has control over it, and to make sure it causes as little inconvenience as possible.

Candidal infection (thrush)
What is it?
Candida albicans is a fungus of the yeast family. This very common microbe is normally found in your digestive tract and is often present in small quantities, on your skin and in your vagina, without causing any ill-effects.

This type of harmless presence is known as colonisation. *Candida* tends to become a problem only if it overgrows – often in people who are already vulnerable.

When *Candida* causes active infection, as opposed to harmless colonisation, it is known as candidiasis or candidosis. The term 'thrush' is usually used for active candidal infections of the mouth or vagina.

Who gets it?
Candidal infection of the mouth can occur in susceptible people of all ages, especially:

- babies

- elderly people with ill-fitting dentures

Candidal infection

This infection is also called thrush and is caused by *Candida albicans*, a fungus of the yeast family. This very common organism is found in your digestive tract and is often present in small quantities on your skin and in your vagina. It usually causes no ill-effects. It tends to become a problem only if it overgrows – often in people who are already vulnerable. The yellow area shows the infected vagina and vulva.

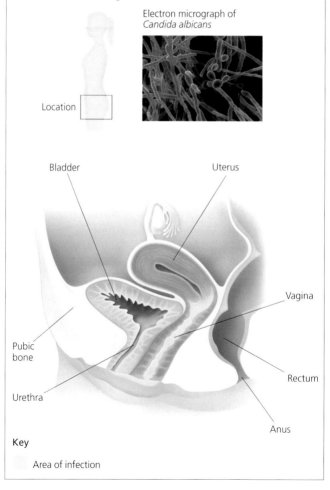

Electron micrograph of *Candida albicans*

Location

Bladder

Uterus

Vagina

Pubic bone

Rectum

Urethra

Anus

Key

Area of infection

- people with pneumonia

- those infected with HIV.

In babies, *Candida* can also cause nappy rash. At any age, it can produce a 'sweat rash' with soreness and redness in skin folds, such as between the male scrotum and thigh area, and under women's breasts. It probably takes hold in these areas because they are warm and wet and have plenty of nutrients for the fungus to grow.

How does it grow?

At any one time, about one in five women has candida colonisation of her vagina. It is kept under control by a delicate balance of bacteria in the vagina, which compete with the yeast for nutrients. Chemicals in your vaginal secretions also keep a check on its growth.

As with BV, thrush occurs when the organism multiplies and displaces much of the normal flora. The yeast normally exists as spores (seed-like, dormant forms) but when it begins to cause disease these spores germinate and grow into microscopic, branching strands of fungus (mycelia).

The mycelia spread over your vaginal walls and burrow into them, causing inflammation. The red, inflamed vaginal walls, covered with a whitish net of mycelia, are said to resemble the breast of a song thrush – hence the common name, 'thrush'. The white, net-like membrane can be scraped off and underneath, in severe cases, the skin may leak minute drops of blood.

Vaginal discharge

Most books describe the vaginal discharge of candidal infection as looking like cottage cheese, and often it is like that. However, the discharge can vary considerably.

Sometimes the secretions are actually drier than normal and often they can be watery, or even contain pus that appears greenish in colour. The abnormal vaginal discharge caused by *Candida* is usually odourless, although you may detect a yeasty or mushroom-like smell.

Inflammation

The inflammation is relatively mild at first, causing itching rather than soreness, but you may become extremely sore if it continues. You can feel the irritation on your vulva but are rarely aware of any sensation within your vagina.

The vulval itching is caused by discharge spilling out over the vulval skin from the relatively insensitive vagina. However, the main pool of infection (the reservoir) remains in your vagina.

Your vulva is red and itchy and, if you scratch it, it quickly becomes sore. A badly affected vulva becomes so inflamed that the skin swells up and the swollen vulval skin develops shallow splits along the folds down each side. This is painful and can get so bad that it makes walking difficult.

As you can imagine, passing urine over such a sore vulva causes a burning sensation. This burning on passing urine is often attributed, wrongly, to a urinary tract infection.

How is it diagnosed?

Active *Candida albicans* can be seen on stained slides of vaginal secretions examined with a microscope. This is the method of diagnosis used in genitourinary medicine clinics.

It is not usually possible in GP surgeries. In a GP surgery, or family planning clinic, candidiasis is confirmed by a sample sent to the local microbiology laboratory.

Your doctor may wait for the result. Alternatively, he or she can make the diagnosis and start treatment on the grounds of your symptoms and examination of your genital area alone.

Candida can also show up on slides taken for cervical smears, but the delay in getting the result of a cervical smear often means that the finding is of academic interest only. You are either better by then, or the diagnosis has been made in some other way and treatment completed.

Often the diagnosis is made because you have bought or been prescribed specific thrush treatment and it has worked.

Is the diagnosis reliable?

One in five women has inactive *Candida* in her vagina. So a positive culture does not prove that it is the cause of the symptoms.

On-the-spot microscopy of a vaginal sample, available at a genitourinary medicine clinic, can help distinguish between active candidal infection, as shown by the presence of growing mycelia, and inactive spores, which may just be passengers. Even if there is evidence of active infection, however, it is still possible that there is more than one cause of your symptoms – for example, you may have candidiasis and genital warts (see page 91).

What are the predisposing factors?

Much has been written about the causes of candidal infection. Most candidiasis occurs out of the blue with no obvious predisposing cause.

Treatment with broad-spectrum antibiotics, such as penicillins, is one of the most common trigger factors. Antibiotics kill bacteria but not yeasts, and the broader the spectrum the more species of bacteria the drug will attack.

If you have taken a course of antibiotics, the number of bacteria in your vagina will be reduced and some, or many, of the types (depending on the broadness of the antibiotic's spectrum) will have been wiped out altogether.

As a result, fewer bacteria are competing with *Candida* for nutrients. This gives the yeast an opportunity to occupy the space left by the bacteria, and it grows out of control, causing an attack of thrush.

Female sex hormones seem to encourage the growth of *Candida* and this accounts for several facts about candidiasis:

- It is common in pregnancy.

- It often occurs in the few days before menstruation.

- It is generally more common during your reproductive years.

These are all times when your oestrogen levels are high.

For a long time, the oral contraceptive pill was also thought to increase the risk of developing candidal infection. There is no evidence for this, however.

It is true that the high-oestrogen pills of the 1960s and 1970s might have increased candidiasis. The contraceptive pills used now probably have too low a hormone content to cause a problem.

Another risk factor for candidal infection is reduced immunity, which may occur if you are:

- on steroid treatment

- receiving cancer chemotherapy

- HIV positive.

Candidiasis is also more common in people with diabetes, particularly if the diabetes is not well controlled. This is because *Candida* thrives in conditions of high sugar content.

What is the treatment?

Candidal infection is self-limiting and will always get better eventually, for example, an attack that begins just before a period often disappears spontaneously when the period starts. However, it can be most unpleasant while it lasts and, with a bad attack, you will not want to wait for nature to take its course.

Antifungal drugs

Although the symptoms of candidiasis are mainly vulval, the treatment is aimed at eradicating the reservoir of yeast that is growing in your vagina. Antifungal drugs of the '-azole' group (such as clotrimazole) are the mainstay of therapy.

These can be used as pessaries or cream inserted into your vagina. Some (such as fluconazole) may be taken as tablets/capsules by mouth.

Cream for external use is available to smear onto the outside of your vulva and this often helps to alleviate symptoms more quickly. Used alone, however, it does not seem to improve the cure rate – presumably because cream on this outer area has no effect on the continuing infection in your vaginal reservoir.

Studies have not shown any convincing difference in effectiveness between any of the drug treatments available – pessaries, vaginal creams or oral tablets, whether available on prescription or over the counter. They all eradicate *Candida* in about 90 per cent of cases.

You may prefer to take the treatment orally because it is more convenient and less messy. On the other hand, you may feel that it is better to apply something directly to the affected area rather than have the drug dispersed throughout your body.

Over-the-counter drugs to treat candidal infection

The two main antifungal drugs used to treat candidal infection are clotrimazole and fluconazole. They are available in many different forms so that you may choose one to suit you. You can buy the following 'over-the-counter' drugs from your pharmacist.

Generic name	Trade (or proprietary) name	Formulation
Clotrimazole	Canesten	Pessary (insertion into vagina)
		Vaginal cream (internal use)
		Cream (external use)
Fluconazole	Diflucan One	Oral capsule
	Canesten Oral	Oral capsule

Whatever treatment is used, symptoms begin to improve within a day or so. Mild irritation may linger for several days.

Removal of predisposing factors

Besides taking the antifungal treatment, it is important to identify and remove, if possible, any predisposing factors. Given the organism's predilection for a warm, wet environment, most experts recommend keeping your genital area as cool and dry as possible by wearing loose, absorbent clothing made of natural products such as cotton.

Almost all the books and leaflets advise trying to reduce the risk of infecting your vagina from your bowel by wiping your anus from front to back after passing a motion. Although there is no firm evidence that this helps, it would seem to be logical advice.

Vaginal douche

You might also try using live, natural 'bio' yoghurt as a vaginal douche. It contains a type of bacterium known as *Lactobacillus*. This type of bacterium is also found in normal vaginas, but is often absent when there is an attack of thrush.

The theory is that replacing the vaginal flora with *Lactobacillus* from live 'bio' yoghurt may help to rebalance the bacterial flora and displace the excess *Candida* causing your attack. Although it is probably not effective in the way suggested, yoghurt is soothing and can be a helpful, if somewhat messy, addition to symptom relief.

Some people recommend taking it by mouth. Although this is probably more pleasant, there is no logic to this.

Anti-candidal diets

There is a vogue for 'anti-candidal diets' and for attributing many symptoms and conditions to a 'yeast problem' – from myalgic encephalitis (ME) through to depression and irritable bowel syndrome. There is no scientific basis for this.

Claims that *Candida* spreads through the body have been shown to be false. It is not found in the bloodstream except when it has been injected by users of brown heroin or in those with terminal leukaemia.

Anti-candidal diets are based on some illogical concepts. These diets usually recommend eradicating most yeast products from your diet. The idea that eradicating one type of yeast from the diet will stop another is most odd, especially when you realise that yeasts are killed along with almost all other micro-organisms by stomach acid soon after swallowing.

However, there are reports of women finding these diets helpful. Provided a healthy nutritional intake can be assured (which in some it cannot), they do no harm.

What about your sexual partner?

Candidal infection is not classed as a sexually transmitted infection, and it is common for virgins to suffer from thrush. It is, however, more likely to develop if you are having frequent, vigorous, sexual intercourse – thrush and cystitis used to be thought of as 'honeymoon' afflictions.

This is from a mechanical cause bringing on an infective one. The act of intercourse can interfere with the vagina's natural defences to infection, for example, by damaging delicate tissues which are then more vulnerable to the ever-present *Candida*.

Candida thrives in a warm, wet, acid environment, preferably high in sugars. For this reason, men do not get severe attacks of thrush because the penis, unlike the vagina, does not normally provide any of these conditions. Instead, men get three, slightly different conditions:

- mild infection

- allergic reaction

- more severe infection in men with diabetes.

Mild infection

The most common is a mild, red speckling of the end of the penis within about 24 hours of intercourse. This represents a short-lived candidal infection.

This infection will disappear spontaneously, provided the man refrains from reinfecting himself through further sexual intercourse with an infected woman – the so-called 'dipstick effect'. Microbiological swab tests taken from the partner's penis around the time of the rash will usually show *Candida*.

Allergic reaction

Another form of male thrush is thought to be an allergic reaction to the woman's infection. In this case, soon after intercourse, the man notices a mild burning on the end of his penis that lasts for an hour or two; the actual candida yeasts cannot usually be detected.

The treatment for both these male manifestations of *Candida* is to treat the woman's infection, and then the man's problem will almost always resolve itself. There is generally no need for him to be treated.

Men with diabetes

The third form of male candidal infection occurs in men with diabetes. The *Candida* feeds and grows on the high levels of sugar from the diabetes. The symptoms are similar to those of the women's condition, with severe itching, soreness and swelling of the foreskin.

It has a typical appearance and diabetes is often diagnosed in men just from this particularly nasty form of thrush, which can also occur in those who are not sexually active. The infection goes when the diabetes is treated.

What about recurrent candidal infection?

It is not uncommon for women to suffer frequent attacks of candidiasis at certain times in their lives. These attacks can be distressing and difficult to control. The problem is probably best tackled in a series of steps:

1 check the diagnosis

2 avoid triggers

3 use preventive treatment

4 check for skin problems.

Check the diagnosis

First, it is essential to confirm that the diagnosis is correct. The list of possible diagnoses is large and includes all the causes of vulval irritation, dysuria and vaginal discharge.

Sometimes you, your partner or your doctor may label sexual problems as recurrent candidal infection. To confirm the diagnosis, you must have had more than one positive test with symptoms present, and at least some response to specific anti-candida treatments.

Avoid triggers

Once the diagnosis has been confirmed, the second step is to search for avoidable trigger factors and change them. General measures (see page 129) should be tried. With unavoidable factors you may still know when your next attack is likely to occur, for example, before your next period or after a romantic weekend.

Use preventive treatment

If your thrush is predictable, the third step is to take some preventive treatment before the onset of an attack. For example, using an antifungal cream as lubrication during intercourse can sometimes prevent attacks that come on after sex. With the medication for candidal infection freely available over the counter, you can experiment and come up with a regimen that suits you.

Some years ago there was a belief that eradicating *Candida* from the bowel would prevent reinfection of the vagina from that source and hence any recurrences. Although this seems a plausible strategy, studies showed no benefit – the bowel quickly becomes reinfected with *Candida* and the vagina soon after.

Even in recurrent candidal infection there is no benefit in treating a male sexual partner. It seems to make no difference.

Check for skin problems

It is thought that recurrent candidal infection in some women takes advantage of skin conditions such as vulval eczema. The skin is already damaged by the eczema, making it more vulnerable to the ever-present *Candida*, which then multiplies in the affected tissue.

The fourth step, therefore, may be to get a dermatological opinion on whether there is a skin problem and, if there is, how to resolve it. After having several attacks some women develop an allergic reaction to *Candida* in their vaginas, which means that even the smallest amount of the yeast (which would not normally be noticed) can trigger a nasty attack of itching and soreness.

If you have this sort of allergic reaction you may find that you have almost permanent symptoms. Obviously you need to be very careful to follow the hygiene rules but they may not be enough.

One of the best ways to deal with this kind of allergic reaction is to reset the allergic response to *Candida*. The aim is to eradicate *Candida* from the vagina altogether for long enough for the allergic process to 'forget' how to react to it.

Weekly doses of clotrimazole pessaries or oral fluconazole (about 100 mg) usually do the trick and stop all symptoms. It is quite safe to take this for three to six months and after stopping most women find that, although they may get the odd attack of thrush, the awful, almost continuous symptoms do not recur.

Trichomoniasis
What is it?
Trichomoniasis is the name given to infection with *Trichomonas vaginalis* (TV). TV is a motile protozoan from the same family of organisms as the amoebae that you may have studied in school.

It is a single cell with an undulating membrane (rather like a flouncy skirt) and five flagella (whip-like structures sticking out of the end). The flagella beat rapidly so that, under a microscope, the organism seems to spin around in a busy way.

It is not a virus, a bacterium or a yeast, but the next grade up in complexity in the microbe world. Unlike the microbes that cause BV or candidal infection, TV does not occur naturally in the vagina.

Where does it come from?

It has to come from elsewhere, almost always from a sexual partner. After sexual exposure to TV the usual incubation period (the time between contact with an infected person and the appearance of symptoms) is 5 to 28 days.

What are the symptoms?

TV usually causes severe inflammation although, like other vaginal infections, there may be no symptoms at all (asymptomatic). However, this asymptomatic state is rare with trichomoniasis.

The typical vaginal discharge of TV contains pus and sometimes blood streaks, and often means that you have to resort to panty liners to protect against constant wetness. The inflammation affects the whole of your vagina and, importantly, the vaginal surface of your cervix.

Your vulva is also affected by the vaginal discharge spilling over it, and becomes sore and red. This may even extend down to your thighs.

The inflammation of your cervix may be so bad that the lab cannot read your cervical smear. It may report just seeing TV on it. A repeat smear will be necessary after treatment for TV.

Trichomoniasis

Trichomoniasis is the name given to infection with *Trichomonas vaginalis* (TV). This is a motile protozoan from the same family of organisms as the amoebae. It is not a virus, a bacterium or a yeast, but the next grade up in complexity in the microbe world. TV does not occur naturally in the vagina and it has to come from elsewhere, almost always from a sexual partner. TV usually generates severe inflammation. The yellow area shows the infected vagina and vulva.

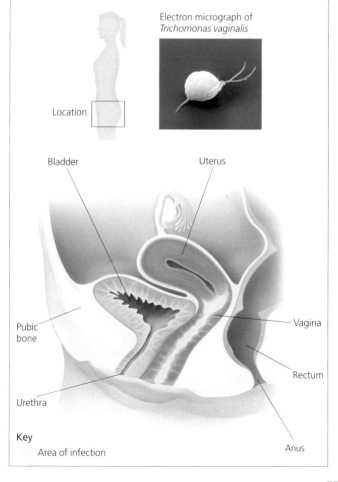

Location

Electron micrograph of *Trichomonas vaginalis*

Bladder

Uterus

Pubic bone

Urethra

Vagina

Rectum

Anus

Key

Area of infection

Why is it important?

Trichomoniasis does not have any long-term consequences or complications. It is important because it is commonly found with more serious infections such as gonorrhoea and chlamydial infection (see page 101). As TV causes symptoms, and gonorrhoea and chlamydial infection usually do not, TV is a trigger to look for the other two infections.

How is it diagnosed?

Trichomonas vaginalis is found in three main ways. Fresh discharge may be swabbed and examined under a microscope in a genitourinary medicine clinic ('on-the-spot' microscopy), which will show the organisms busily moving around. They may also be cultured from a vaginal swab sent to the laboratory (by a GP, for example) or unsuspected TV may occasionally be seen on a routine cervical smear (see above).

Is the diagnosis reliable?

No test for TV is more than about 70 per cent accurate. A number of factors complicate the diagnosis.

If it is seen on culture or 'on-the-spot' microscopy, the diagnosis is seldom wrong. However, there may be too few organisms to be seen or, if the specimen has been taken at some distance from the laboratory, the organisms may die in transit.

If TV has been found only on a cervical smear, it may have been confused with some types of immune cell (which it can resemble once stained with dyes as part of the cervical smear process). The diagnosis has to remain dubious until it can be confirmed in another way.

Often TV is present together with the bacteria that cause BV and, because the latter are easier to find, BV may be the only diagnosis made. Fortunately, treatment for BV works for trichomoniasis too.

If trichomoniasis is not diagnosed, however, your male partner will not realise that he needs to be treated and you may catch it back from him. Failing to diagnose trichomoniasis also means a missed opportunity to look for and treat any accompanying infections, such as chlamydial infection and gonorrhoea.

What are the predisposing factors?

As TV is sexually transmitted, the predisposing factors are all those that increase the risk of catching any STI. Studies have shown that the following factors are more common in people with an STI:

- A recent change in sexual partner

- Sex outside a relationship

- Being aged under 20 years

- Living in an inner city

- Not using barrier contraceptive methods (for example, condoms).

What is the treatment?

The drug treatment for trichomoniasis is the narrow-spectrum antibiotic, metronidazole (see page 58), which is given orally. Symptoms improve very quickly, within a couple of days. The gel form, which is an option for treating BV, is not as effective as tablets for killing TV.

If the treatment doesn't appear to work, it can be for three reasons. The most common is that you have been reinfected. You should make sure that your partner has been treated – preferably at a genitourinary medicine (GUM) clinic.

Two other rare reasons are because you have a strain of TV that is resistant to metronidazole, or the antibiotic has not been absorbed in sufficient quantities to kill the bacteria. If treatment does not seem to work, you should see a GUM specialist. Your partner also needs to be seen again and you both may need another type of antibiotic treatment.

Vaginal infections and their treatments

There are three main vaginal infections. Their different characteristics and treatments are listed below.

Condition	Symptoms	Treatment	Comment
Bacterial vaginosis (BV)	Fishy odour; little or no irritation	Metronidazole; clindamycin cream	Very common; worse after sex
Candidal infection (thrush)	White discharge; itching, leading to soreness	Antifungals (pessaries or tablets)	Worse with antibiotics
Tricho-moniasis	Soreness; watery discharge	Metronidazole	Sexually transmitted

What about your sexual partner?

Trichomonas vaginalis can survive on objects such as sex toys, and even lavatory seats, for up to 45 minutes. There has also been a report of the infection being transmitted in a jacuzzi.

However, studies of women who have developed trichomoniasis almost always find that it has been sexually transmitted. If you have trichomoniasis, your male partner will carry the organism for a few weeks after your last sexual encounter. However, as with candidal infection, the organism will eventually die in a man unless he is reinfected.

Testing a man for TV is unsatisfactory. Occasionally, the organism can be seen but tests usually show nothing, or just 'non-specific' inflammation of the male urethra. Unfortunately, non-specific inflammation in men is labelled non-specific urethritis (NSU), a condition usually caused by *Chlamydia*, or related bacteria, and requiring quite different treatment.

It is, therefore, important that your male partner sees an experienced GUM doctor to sort out this complex situation and it is essential that your partner's doctor is aware of your diagnosis. Regardless of what is found (or not found) on examination, your male partner must be treated for trichomoniasis if you have it, or reinfection is likely to occur.

If your partner is female, she should be checked by a doctor, too. This is because TV is easily transmitted from woman to woman on sex toys and fingers.

Trichomoniasis often occurs with gonorrhoea and chlamydial infection. For this reason it is essential that you and your partner are also examined for these more serious conditions.

What about recurrent trichomoniasis?

If trichomoniasis comes back after you are sure that it has been killed, you must have been reinfected, most probably from your sexual partner. It does not return of its own accord.

Therefore, before assuming that the condition has come back it is important to make sure that the original and subsequent diagnoses were correct. With a true recurrence, it is important to tell the difference between reinfection and failure of the treatment.

Genital herpes simplex infection
What is it?

A high percentage of the adult population carries the herpes simplex virus (HSV). Most commonly, it affects the lips of susceptible individuals, where it is called a cold sore.

Most people infected with the virus do not go on to develop cold sores, and in these people the virus merely lies dormant. HSV can also affect the genital area where, again, it is dormant in most of the 10 to 15 per cent or so of the adult population who are affected.

There are two types of virus: HSV-1 and HSV-2. Until a few years ago, type 1 was almost entirely confined to the mouth, with type 2 affecting the genitals. However, this has now changed: both can be found commonly in either site – probably because more people are having oral sex than previously. You might have read that it is important to know which type of virus you have because type 1 is less likely to recur than type 2.

Herpes simplex virus infection

A high percentage of the adult population carries the herpes simplex virus (HSV). Most commonly it affects the lips of susceptible individuals, where it is called a cold sore. HSV can also affect the genital area, where it is dormant in most of the 10–15 per cent of the adult population who are infected. The area of the infected vulva is shown, with a portion enlarged to show the appearance in detail.

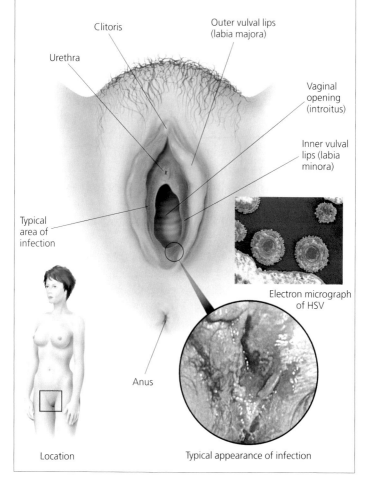

Clitoris

Urethra

Outer vulval lips (labia majora)

Vaginal opening (introitus)

Inner vulval lips (labia minora)

Typical area of infection

Electron micrograph of HSV

Anus

Location

Typical appearance of infection

How do you get it?

Herpes infection of the mouth and lips tends to be contracted during childhood from other children. Genital herpes, however, is usually caught from a sexual partner in adult life.

Transmission may occur from your partner's genitals during vaginal sex, or from his or her lips during oral sex. Many people become infected with HSV without ever knowing it. They either have no symptoms or have some mild soreness, which they attribute to thrush or some other condition.

The incubation period (the time from infection to symptoms) is roughly five days. Herpes is a recurrent infection, but the first attack (technically known as the initial or primary attack) is usually the worst.

What are the symptoms?

An initial attack may begin as a flu-like illness with aching in your back or down your legs, and a tingling at the site of entry of the virus. This illness – a type of warning sign – is called a prodrome.

After a day or two, the lymph glands in your groin become enlarged and tender, and painful blisters begin to develop on your genitals. In due course, these blisters burst leaving several small, exquisitely painful ulcers.

In the worst attacks, blisters continue to appear for two to three weeks before healing starts. After this, you remain infected with HSV, and the disease will follow one of three courses:

1   You may never get another attack and the virus may become completely dormant.
2   You may suffer one or more recurrences, weeks or

months later. These recurrences are likely to be milder and shorter than the initial attack.

3   You may have no further symptoms but occasionally you may shed sufficient numbers of the virus to infect your partner even when you do not have active sores. This process is known as asymptomatic shedding. You get no more symptoms but can infect others.

Asymptomatic shedding

As you can be infectious without symptoms, about 50 per cent of new attacks of HSV occur in people in stable relationships. Presumably, the partner was unaware that he or she ever had herpes and was an asymptomatic shedder at the time of transmission.

Asymptomatic shedding is not very common. Most people with herpes know when they are infectious because they develop symptoms every time. However, it is a possibility and throws up two main worries:

1   If you are an asymptomatic shedder, you can't know when you are infectious and so can't avoid having intercourse at that time and risk infecting your partner. This can have an understandably serious effect on your sex life – you may worry each time you have intercourse about transmitting the infection.

2   If you or your partner suddenly develops herpes in a stable relationship it is probably because the other partner is an asymptomatic shedder – but it can raise niggling doubts that one of you might have been recently infected through intercourse with someone else. Such doubts can become pervasive and even destroy relationships.

How is it diagnosed?

Current tests for HSV rely on finding the virus. The tests are quite specialised and are usually done only at a GUM clinic, although they can be done by some GPs.

Looking for the virus

A positive result shows up only on samples taken from fresh blisters or sores. Tests have to go to the laboratory and, depending on test used, results take a week or more to come back. Severe herpes is too nasty to wait this long and so treatment is started before confirmation from the laboratory.

Looking for antibodies

There are blood tests that look for HSV antibodies. These are proteins made by white blood cells to attack the virus.

These tests can show whether you have ever been infected with HSV. However, as they are not 100% accurate, they tend to be used mainly for research purposes.

These antibody tests are not currently funded by the NHS, but your GUM clinic may be able to arrange for you to have one. Studies using these tests show that up to 15 per cent of British women have antibodies to genital herpes, which is far more than ever knew they were even at risk.

Is the diagnosis reliable?

Like many women, you may only ever get mild attacks of herpes and find the symptoms hard to differentiate from those of candidiasis. Indeed, it is likely that many symptoms attributed to recurrent candidal infections are, in fact, attacks of herpes virus infection.

False-negative results

A swab test for HSV can be negative even though the condition is present. Such false-negative results are common in herpes infections.

They occur for several reasons. It may be that:

- your sores are beginning to heal and no longer shed the virus

- you have already had treatment for herpes

- the samples are not handled in the proper way before they get to the laboratory.

Positive for antibodies but not infectious

The blood test for antibodies to HSV, by contrast, can be positive even if you are not having a herpes attack. It shows that you have been infected by HSV at some time, but it does not prove that a sore is caused by herpes or indicate anything about your infectiousness.

Case history: David

David, a 30-year-old office manager, developed symptoms of an initial attack of genital herpes. His partner, Nicola, who had no history of herpes, appeared to have given it to him (as there was no other sexual partner involved).

It seemed possible, therefore, that she was an asymptomatic shedder and had passed the infection on to David in complete innocence. Nicola's GP and practice nurse showed her pictures of the herpes blisters and, along with discussions with other herpes sufferers, she soon learned to recognise symptoms of herpes.

Six months later Nicola was confident enough to realise that she had been having herpes attacks all along. As they were so mild she had mistaken them for thrush.

What are the predisposing factors?

Your first attack of genital herpes will be acquired sexually. The frequency and severity of recurrences depend on many factors, mainly related to your immune status.

Stress

Frequently you will be able to relate attacks to stress in your life – for example, exams, getting married, moving house. You may get attacks just before your periods, which can easily be confused with attacks of candidal infection, because *Candida* also prefers the time before a period to attack.

Sunlight

If you also get cold sores, you know that sunlight brings them on. Similarly, the sun can trigger genital herpes, especially if you expose the area that usually develops herpes by sunbathing naked or in a very brief swimsuit.

Low immunity

If you are an asymptomatic carrier, the first attack that you notice could occur years after you caught the virus. This may happen if you get severely run down, or if your immunity is very low, for example, as a result of having cancer chemotherapy or if you have HIV infection.

What is the treatment?

Specific drugs against the herpes virus are safe, effective and very rarely cause side effects. Aciclovir (Zovirax), valaciclovir (Valtrex) and famciclovir (Famvir) are available on prescription.

There is no convincing difference in the effectiveness of each drug, although the number of daily doses varies between them. You only have to take valaciclovir and famciclovir once and twice daily, respectively, but have to take aciclovir five times a day. However, aciclovir is currently the cheapest and is, therefore, the most frequently prescribed.

All these drugs start to improve symptoms within 48 hours and they can all suppress further attacks while you are still taking them – so people with frequent recurrences may be offered a course of suppressive treatment.

None, however, has any proven long-term effect. After stopping an anti-herpes drug, the risk of an attack is probably the same as if the infection had been left to take its natural course.

These treatments are therefore not a cure as such but they do relieve symptoms. They can also prevent the virus emerging and so, while you are taking them, they can prevent you passing herpes on.

Are there any complications?

There are no long-term physical effects. The main problem with herpes infection is the effect that fear of transmission can have on current and future relationships. If you have herpes you have a big dilemma about what and when to tell your sexual partner.

This is especially a problem if you are starting a new relationship. If you tell him very early in the relationship, before you have intercourse, it may blight your budding romance.

If you tell him when the relationship is more established or, worse, if you infect him before you tell him, he may feel angry that you didn't warn him sooner. Most men worthy of you, however, will be understanding when you explain that you can protect them reasonably well from catching it by avoiding attack times and using condoms.

Risk of infecting your baby

The medical risk is that of passing the infection to your baby at birth. If you have an active herpes sore when you go into labour, there is a chance that the baby could pick up the infection as he or she passes through the birth canal.

Some obstetricians used to recommend a caesarean section for such circumstances. However, it is very rare for a baby to become infected.

In any case the baby can be treated safely and effectively with the drug that you are taking, although there is a risk that it might then carry the infection. Caesarean deliveries are no longer recommended just because you have herpes.

What about your sexual partner?

One of the main worries that you may have with a new diagnosis of HSV is 'Where did it come from?'. It is not always possible to find visual evidence of HSV (such as sores) on a partner, even if he or she was the source of the infection. So, until recently, it has been difficult to say who infected whom.

However, there are now blood tests to help detect whether your partner is immune to HSV. If he is immune, he must have previously been infected with HSV.

In this case, it is likely that either your partner was the source of the infection or you have already passed your infection to him. On the other hand, if he is not immune, your partner could not have been the source and is still at risk of catching herpes from you.

HSV is an STI. As STIs tend to be found together, it is advisable for both you and your partner to get checked for any other STIs (such as chlamydial infection or gonorrhoea) that may be present without causing obvious symptoms.

What about recurrent HSV infection?

Recurrences (repeated infections) occur in about 50 per cent of people after the initial attack. They are often preceded by a prodrome – a collection of symptoms such as shooting twinge-like pains down the legs or back followed by tingling or pain at the site where the blisters break out.

The actual recurrent outbreaks are usually similar to the initial attack, but milder and are less and less severe and frequent as time goes by. There are three ways that anti-herpes drugs can be used to help recurrences:

1 As soon as you develop an attack of herpes, you can take a five-day course of an anti-herpes drug, which, if taken soon enough, may reduce the length and severity of the attack. Studies have shown, however, that, if your attack lasts for five or fewer days, taking an anti-herpes drug once it has begun does not appreciably shorten the attack or the infectious period.
2 The drugs are more likely to be effective if you are able to predict the onset of an attack, either because you know what triggers it or because you recognise the warning signs (the prodrome). If you can start treatment before the attack has really begun, you can sometimes stop it progressing to the blister stage altogether – so-called 'abortive therapy'.

3 You can take anti-herpes drugs continuously. If your attacks are very frequent and disruptive to your life, you can take the anti-herpes medication daily on a long-term basis to prevent the herpes breaking out (continuous suppressive therapy). This is taken in a lower dose than that used for attacks.

Case history: Monique

Monique, a 21-year-old nurse, had suffered from genital herpes for two years. Her attacks occurred every four months and more frequently when she was under stress.

She was arranging her wedding and was looking forward to a honeymoon in the sun. However, she feared that both the stress of the arrangements and the effect of lots of sex and sun might trigger a herpes attack on her honeymoon.

Her GP prescribed a one-month course of aciclovir to suppress her attacks – this was to be taken twice daily from the week before the wedding. She had a lovely 'big day' and a herpes-free honeymoon.

For most people, herpes attacks are a minor inconvenience. If you are in this group, you should try where possible to avoid precipitating factors (such as stress) and bathe the area in a salt solution (see page 127) whenever you have an attack.

Aciclovir cream

Aciclovir is also available over the counter from pharmacies in cream form. Although studies have not shown any benefit from using creams, many women are convinced that it helps them, so it may be worth a try. Strictly speaking, however, it is licensed only for sale over the counter for use on lip cold sores.

How herpes is spread

Herpes is passed on by direct contact of infected sores with uninfected skin. This skin usually has to be thin, such as that on the lips or genitals, to allow the virus to settle in and grow.

It is therefore nearly always passed only by contact between two people's genitals during intercourse or from mouth to genitals during oral sex.

It is possible, but uncommon, to transfer your own herpes to another part of your body, for example, if you touch your cold sores on your lips and then immediately afterwards touch your genitals. The virus is destroyed by soap and water and therefore, if you have got it on your hands by touching a sore, spread can be prevented by simple handwashing.

There is no risk of casual social transmission. It is not transmitted on towels, in swimming baths, on cups or on glasses.

Genital warts
What are they?

Genital warts are caused by sexually transmitted strains of the human papilloma virus (HPV). There are over 100 different strains of HPV. Many of them cause warts on other parts of the body such as the hands and the feet (where they are the cause of verrucas).

Genital warts are distinct from those elsewhere on the body. The genital wart virus types are confined to the genital area and the non-genital types are not found on the genitals.

How common are they?

Genital HPV is a very common infection. It is said that approximately 30 per cent of sexually active people will have had HPV infection at some time although the vast majority will never have had actual warts.

These people will be clear of the infection, without ever realising that they had it, two to three years after catching it. As carriers of HPV during this time they may, however, be infectious and able to spread HPV to their partner(s).

What are the warts like?

The strains of genital wart viruses can be divided into two types: those that are benign and those that have been linked with cancer (oncogenic). The benign strains irritate the skin of the vulva, which responds by growing more than usual, forming little piles of skin (warts) containing a scattering of virus particles.

Genital warts appear rather like tiny, pale-pink growths on the vulva. The oncogenic strains (those thought to cause cancer) mainly affect the cervix and can cause cervical cancer; normally, the only sign of infection with this type is an abnormal cervical smear. The warts that you can see on your vulva are therefore not those that increase the risk of cancer.

The wart virus gains entry through the minute cuts or splits in your skin that are often present; the main sites are the lower part towards the back of your vulva and around your anus. The virus then spreads widely through your genital skin, causing warts to pop up at random rather like mushrooms in a field.

Do they cause problems?

Warts are a cosmetic problem. If they grow big and trap bacteria in their crevices, they may itch.

As with any other STIs, they can also affect relationships. Their incubation period is long, up to

Genital warts

Genital warts are caused by sexually transmitted strains of the human papilloma virus (HPV). Most of those infected show no symptoms at all and the infection goes away spontaneously after two or three years. During this time most of them will be carriers of HPV and may be infectious, but will not be aware of this. The area of the infected vulva is shown, with a portion enlarged to show the appearance in detail.

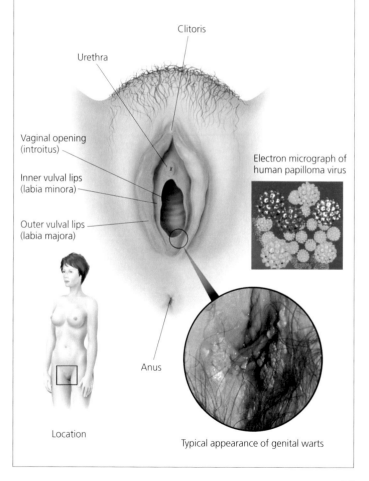

Clitoris

Urethra

Vaginal opening (introitus)

Inner vulval lips (labia minora)

Outer vulval lips (labia majora)

Electron micrograph of human papilloma virus

Anus

Location

Typical appearance of genital warts

Genital warts in men

Genital warts are reported more frequently by men than by women, probably because they are more visible on the penis. The inset shows the warts in more detail.

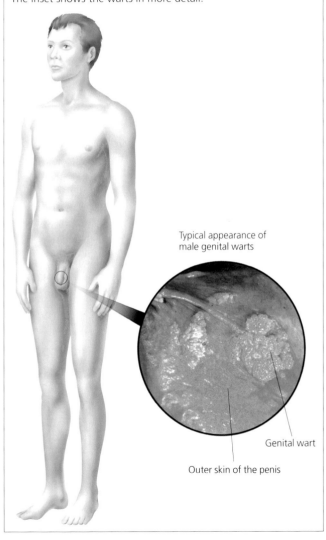

Typical appearance of male genital warts

Genital wart

Outer skin of the penis

several months, and if they arise anew in a fairly long-term partnership they may sow doubts and mistrust about fidelity.

How are they diagnosed?

There are no commonly available tests for genital warts and the diagnosis relies on the doctor or nurse recognising them on examination. The diagnosis can be proved by surgical removal and examination of a specimen (a biopsy), but this is rather a drastic step under normal circumstances.

In the future, there will be tests for the presence of the virus, but current work is aimed at developing tests to detect the cancer-causing (oncogenic) strains, not the benign ones, for obvious reasons. If you have genital warts you may be at risk for other STIs and should get checked for these too.

Is the diagnosis reliable?

Many blemishes can look like warts. There are skin tags, moles, a viral infection called molluscum contagiosum and many more. It is sometimes advisable to wait and see how a small spot or lump develops – whether it grows and becomes more recognisable, or whether it disappears, as an infected spot might.

Warts generally grow larger or disappear over time. A wart that remains unchanged may not be a wart. If your doctor is in doubt, he or she may suggest a biopsy.

What are the predisposing factors?

To become infected with genital warts you must be (or have been) sexually active, or at least in close intimate contact with someone. HPV infection, even more than herpes, is affected by your immunity.

When your immunity is lowered during pregnancy genital warts can grow quite large. They can become troublesome but they nearly always go of their own accord after the baby is born.

Examples of other immune conditions when warts are more difficult to eradicate are if you have diabetes or systemic lupus erythematosus (SLE), or if you are taking steroid drugs or on kidney dialysis. Warts even seem to be worsened by the normal stresses of day-to-day living.

What is the treatment?

HPV infection is difficult to treat because the virus tends to lie dormant in the body, just like the herpes virus. The best you can hope for is to get rid of the visible warts, not the virus, within the skin; the virus will go in its own good time.

There is still some sense in trying to do this because the visible warts are probably the main sites from which the virus is shed and so removing them may make you less infectious. They are also, of course, the only outward sign of the infection and, as such, are a cosmetic nuisance, so removing them often has a psychological benefit.

There are a vast number of methods for treating warts. This says a lot: if a really successful method existed, all the others would have been abandoned. Treatments aim to do a variety of things.

Drug treatment

Some treatments try to stop the growth of warts by interfering in the growth of the skin cells (an example of this is a plant extract, podophyllin – active ingredient podophyllotoxin – which is marketed as a cream).

Treatments for genital warts

Genital warts are self-limiting and will usually disappear with time. There are a large number of treatments for warts. Those shown are heat treatment, chemical treatment and freezing.

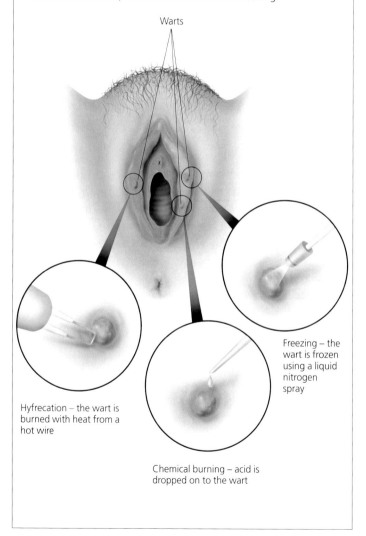

Warts

Freezing – the wart is frozen using a liquid nitrogen spray

Hyfrecation – the wart is burned with heat from a hot wire

Chemical burning – acid is dropped on to the wart

Burning or freezing

Other treatments destroy the warts physically by chemical burning (for example, by using concentrated acid), by burning them with heat (for example, using a hot wire as with hyfrecation) or by freezing them (for example, using liquid nitrogen spray).

Immune stimulation

The newest approach tries to stimulate your immune system to attack the virus – a drug called imiquimod is applied as a cream to stimulate local immunity against the wart virus.

Where do I get treatment?

Some of these treatments may be available in your GP practice, but the GUM clinic is likely to have a greater range of options and will be able to advise you about which are best for your warts. It is likely nowadays that you will be given treatments to apply yourself.

How effective is treatment?

Warts are self-limiting and will usually disappear in time but it can take months or even years for this to happen. The results of treatment vary a great deal from person to person.

Sometimes, one treatment is enough to get rid of the warts. You may find that, although individual warts go away with treatment, new ones pop up elsewhere. Rarely, some warts do not seem to respond at all to therapy and may need to be surgically removed.

Is there a vaccine?

A vaccine against HPV has recently been developed and will be offered to young girls and women to help protect them against certain types of HPV thought to cause many cases of cervical cancer and genital warts.

It is best given before they become sexually active. As the vaccine does not prevent all types of cervical cancer it is important for a women to continue her regular smear tests after she has been vaccinated.

What about your sexual partner?
As most carriers of the genital wart virus do not have warts, your sexual partner may not have visible warts. Warts are associated with other STIs, so it is still worth your partner (as well as you) having a check-up.

Treatments for genital warts

Genital warts are difficult to treat and so there is a wide choice of treatment available. The main ones are listed below.

Drug treatments
- Podophyllotoxin cream/liquid (Warticon)
- Podophyllin paint

Physical treatments
- Freezing, e.g. liquid nitrogen spray
- Chemical burning, e.g. trichloroacetic acid
- Burning, e.g. hyfrecation
- Surgical removal

Immune stimulation, e.g. imiquimod cream (Aldara)

Can skin warts infect the genitals?

You or your partner may wonder whether the warts could have been transmitted from hands or other parts of the body during foreplay. This is very unlikely because skin warts are different from genital warts and each strain of the virus tends to settle only in the areas for which it is specially adapted.

Avoiding cross-infection

It is hard for couples to know what to do about preventing sexual transmission of the virus when one of them has warts and the other does not. In most cases, the other partner is already infected, even though he or she doesn't have actual warts.

Often, the warts have developed in a relationship in which unprotected intercourse has occurred for some time. If so it is highly likely that your partner has already been exposed to your wart virus before either of you realised it. Either that, or your partner may have been the source of the infection in the first place.

If it is unlikely that your partner was the source of the infection and he or she is unlikely to be infected already (for example, if you have not started having intercourse yet or if you have used condoms consistently), it is sensible to try to avoid cross-infection. In this circumstance, you should abstain from intercourse or use condoms until you can be sure that your warts have gone. However, warts frequently recur because the virus remains in your body.

Anyway, there may be a high probability that your partner has already been, or will be, exposed to this benign condition, at some time in the future. You and your partner therefore need to decide between you what steps, if any, you take to try to avoid cross-infection.

What about recurrent genital warts?

It is common for warts to recur after they have been successfully treated, usually within a few months of the previous ones disappearing. This recurrence is not thought to indicate that you have been reinfected by your partner – it is more likely that the virus in your skin has once more begun to thrive.

Currently, nothing can prevent this from happening, except to address any predisposing factors, and then to treat the warts again. Most people are somewhat reassured by studies showing that recurrent warts, on average, do resolve more quickly than the original ones.

Chlamydial infection and gonorrhoea
What are they?

Chlamydia trachomatis and *Neisseria gonorrhoeae*, the bacteria that cause chlamydial infection and gonorrhoea, respectively, have a lot in common. They are both sexually transmitted bacteria that infect your cervix, causing few symptoms.

They both have the potential to spread into your upper genital tract and to cause pelvic inflammatory disease (PID – see page 105). If the bacteria are present on your cervix during childbirth, they can also infect the eyes of your newborn baby, causing conjunctivitis.

The two organisms do, however, have some differences. Chlamydial infection tends to be milder, has a longer incubation period and requires a longer course of treatment. It is also much more common than gonorrhoea, affecting about three per cent of all women who attend family planning clinics, and up to one in ten young women who live in inner city areas.

Gonorrhoea is also known as 'the clap' or 'a dose'. It is an old-fashioned venereal disease which, interestingly, is still a legal ground for divorce in this country. If a woman gets gonorrhoea from her husband, even if he caught it before they were married, she can divorce him – and vice versa!

How are they diagnosed?

There is rarely any sign that you have either infection. Even when looked at through a speculum (see page 119), your cervix may appear normal.

What suggests that you are infected?

Infection may be discovered in other ways:

- In routine tests during treatment for another STI

- Because a partner has symptoms

- Because there are signs of infection on a cervical smear

- Because, after a vaginal birth, an infected woman's newborn baby develops conjunctivitis.

Cervical swabs

Tests are aimed at finding the organisms involved. *Chlamydia trachomatis* and *Neisseria gonorrhoeae* are both detected from a swab taken from the cervix, using a speculum to help the doctor or nurse take a sample from exactly the right place.

New tests

Other new methods have been developed for detecting these infections. These make it possible to detect bacteria both from a swab from your vulva and from a

Infection with *Chlamydia trachomatis* or *Neisseria gonorrhoeae*

Chlamydia trachomatis and *Neisseria gonorrhoeae* infect the cervix. They both have the potential to spread into your upper genital tract and to cause pelvic inflammatory disease.

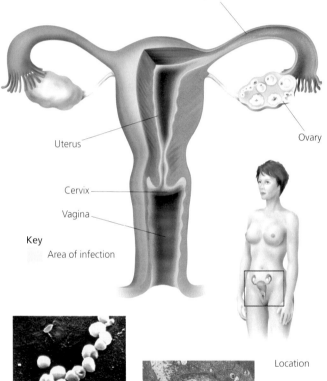

Fallopian tube

Uterus

Ovary

Cervix

Vagina

Key

Area of infection

Location

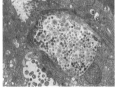

Electron micrograph of *Neisseria gonorrhoeae*

Electron micrograph of *Chlamydia trachomatis*

urine sample alone, without the need for an internal examination. This allows people to take their own specimens if they wish.

Is the diagnosis reliable?

It is hard to say with confidence that any test currently available can completely rule out the presence of *Neisseria gonorrhoeae* or *Chlamydia trachomatis*. *Neisseria gonorrhoeae* bacteria are fragile and are liable to die in the culture before the microbiologist can confirm the diagnosis, especially if the specimen has to be transported some distance to the laboratory.

Even in the best hands, one swab for gonorrhoea will pick up only about 80 per cent of cases. A negative swab for gonorrhoea therefore cannot rule out the diagnosis.

Chlamydia trachomatis is equally difficult to detect. Some methods of detection are better than others. The new test can pick up about 40 per cent more cases than the old test. Even so, especially if it is done on urine, it does not pick up all infected cases.

What is the treatment?

The right antibiotic (see box on page 106) coupled with treatment of your partner should clear these infections. Gonorrhoea is easy to treat and is usually sensitive to a wide range of antibiotics, although resistance to some of these is becoming a problem.

Chlamydial infection is trickier, because only a small range of antibiotics can kill the responsible bacterium. For example, the commonly used penicillin and cephalosporin families of antibiotics (which includes amoxicillin and cephalexin) do not work on *Chlamydia* because they kill bacteria by puncturing the bacterial cell walls – and *Chlamydia trachomatis* doesn't have a cell wall.

Chlamydia species is also able to resist antibiotics for a few days by going into a dormant state. Killing it requires at least seven days of exposure to the correct antibiotic. There is now an antibiotic against *Chlamydia*, azithromycin, which can be taken as a single dose because it lingers in the body for up to three weeks.

Are there any complications?
The most serious complication of both infections is PID. It is estimated that about 10 per cent of women with gonorrhoea have signs of PID, and the risk of developing PID increases as long as the infection goes untreated.

Pelvic inflammatory disease
What is it?
Although it can vary a good deal, the actual progress of the gonorrhoea or chlamydial infection to PID is the same. These infections spread from your cervix up into your uterus and along your fallopian tubes, causing inflammation.

As this inflammation develops, the lining of your fallopian tubes becomes swollen and scarred, and the walls become distorted and stuck together. Over time, the passage down which a fertilised egg should pass becomes blocked.

What are the symptoms?
At first you feel vague pain in your pelvis. You may notice deep pain on intercourse, which may be bad enough to stop you having sex. Depending on the severity of the infection, you may become generally unwell. The most severe pain requires admission to hospital and antibiotics given through a drip.

Comparison of gonorrhoea and chlamydial infection

Chlamydia trachomatis and *Neisseria gonorrhoeae*, the bacteria that cause chlamydial infection and gonorrhoea, respectively, have a lot in common. They are both sexually transmitted bacteria that infect your cervix, causing few or no symptoms.

Characteristic	Gonorrhoea	Chlamydial infection
Incubation period	5–7 days	1–3 weeks
Main site of infection	Cervix	Cervix
Main complication	Pelvic inflammatory disease	Pelvic inflammatory disease
Possible symptoms in the man (sometimes asymptomatic)	Urethral discharge	Urethral discharge
Possible symptoms in the woman (usually asymptomatic)	Vaginal discharge	Vaginal discharge
Association with other infections	Trichomoniasis and/or chlamydial infection	Trichomoniasis and/or gonorrhoeal infection
Common treatments	Amoxicillin (Amoxil) Ciprofloxacin (Ciproxin)	Doxycycline (Vibramycin) Azithromycin (Zithromax)

Less severe, grumbling pain may last for weeks or months and is often diagnosed incorrectly at first because it is hard to place the actual origin of the symptoms. The mildest form of PID produces so little in the way of symptoms that you may be unaware that you ever had it, until, that is, you are told that your fallopian tubes are blocked as a result.

What are the risks?

Infertility is a serious consequence of PID, as is the increased risk of having an ectopic pregnancy. Ectopic pregnancy occurs when an already fertilised egg is halted in its tracks, and prevented from passing into the uterus by the scarring from PID.

The fertilised egg grows in the tube at the point where it lodges. At about six weeks of pregnancy, it can rupture out of the tube, causing sudden, severe, internal bleeding that is life threatening.

Spread to other parts of the genital tract

Neisseria gonorrhoeae and *Chlamydia trachomatis* also cause severe infections elsewhere in the genital tract. They can both cause infections in the glands that lubricate the vulva.

The largest of these, and therefore the most common to get infected, is Bartholin's gland. The condition is known as bartholinitis, if the gland is just inflamed, and Bartholin's abscess if it is filled with pus. The latter usually requires surgery to drain the abscess.

What about your sexual partner?

Both infections may cause a discharge from the penis. Gonorrhoea is more likely to produce noticeable symptoms such as a discharge or pain on passing urine.

Infertility as a result of pelvic inflammatory disease

Infertility can be a consequence of pelvic inflammatory disease (PID) because the fallopian tubes can become blocked. This also increases the risk of an ectopic pregnancy when a fertilised egg is unable to pass through the fallopian tubes. The egg grows in the tube and can rupture.

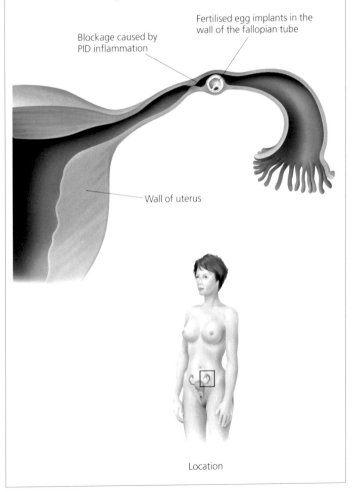

Fertilised egg implants in the wall of the fallopian tube

Blockage caused by PID inflammation

Wall of uterus

Location

So, men with gonorrhoea are more likely to realise that they have an infection than men with chlamydial infection. Indeed, some men with chlamydial infection have no symptoms or signs of it even after special tests at a GUM clinic.

For lesbians the risk of transmitting gonorrhoea or chlamydial infection is much less than if a man is involved. However, as the consequences of either infection can be so serious, it is still advisable for female sexual partners to be checked. Even if the tests are negative both partners may decide to have treatment as a safeguard.

What about recurrent gonorrhoea and chlamydial infection?

Provided that the infections have been adequately treated, there should be no risk of them returning, unless you are reinfected by the same or another sexual partner.

Other causes of pelvic pain

Other things that cause pain in the upper genital tract are:

- endometriosis

- bleeding into or twisting of fibroids or ovarian cysts.

Endometriosis
What is it?

This is a condition in which the columnar epithelium lining of the uterus (endometrium) spreads and grows outside the uterus itself. It is often found stuck on to the inside of the pelvis or the ovaries. Outside the uterus it behaves in the same way as inside, so it continues to build up during the menstrual cycle until the period, when it breaks down and bleeds.

What are the symptoms?

If you have endometriosis you may be quite unaware of it and suffer no inconvenience from it; however, it can be painful. The pain is caused by the pressure of the growing tissue leading up to the period and then from blood being released into the pelvis from the tissue when the period starts.

Pain from endometriosis classically starts just before a period and tails off a day or so after it starts. In the long term, endometriosis can cause scarring, making intercourse painful, blocking the fallopian tubes and causing infertility.

What is the treatment?

If you need treatment, you are likely to be prescribed hormones, similar to the combined oral contraceptive pill, and the symptoms usually improve. Pregnancy may temporarily help the endometriosis but it may return after the pregnancy when menstruation restarts.

Fibroids
What are they?

These are knots of muscle in the wall of the uterus that may stay within the wall, stick out into the cavity of the uterus or project from its outer wall. Many women in their reproductive years have fibroids.

The older you are the more likely you are to have them. However, they tend to shrink after the menopause.

What are the symptoms?

If you do have fibroids the chances are that you will be unaware of them, although your doctor may notice them during a routine pelvic examination. However, if you have fibroids sticking into the uterine cavity, they increase its surface area and make it irregular. This causes increased bleeding and pain during menstruation and sometimes reduces your fertility.

Fibroids can also grow out on short stalks from the uterus and then they may twist and cut off their own blood supply. You might also start to bleed into one of your fibroids, especially if you are pregnant.

What is the treatment?

Twisting or bleeding tends to cause a sudden, very severe pain and you might need admission to hospital. However, once the diagnosis is made you would probably need painkillers only while it settles down by itself.

Ovarian cysts

It is normal to have small ovarian cysts that fluctuate in size during the menstrual cycle. However, sometimes a single cyst can grow large and, similar to a fibroid, twist, cut off its own blood supply or start to bleed into its cavity.

You will feel a sudden onset of pain on one side or the other of your pelvis. It does not usually require treatment and the problem usually resolves by itself.

Ectopic pregnancy

This is a life-threatening condition where a fertilised egg becomes stuck in a fallopian tube and grows there. At about six to eight weeks of pregnancy, the growing embryo can rupture out of the tube and cause severe bleeding into the abdomen. This has to be treated by an emergency operation to stop the bleeding.

Sorting out pelvic pain

The best way to detect what is causing your pelvic pain is for a surgeon to perform a procedure, called a laparoscopy. This usually involves a general anaesthetic.

A small telescope-like tube is then put through a cut in your belly button and air is pumped in. The surgeon can then look down the laparoscope to see what is going on. Even in this situation the surgeon may still not be able to be certain what is wrong.

It is important to remember that pain may be coming from some other organ in your pelvis and be nothing to do with your genital tract. There is more on pelvic pain in the chapter 'What can go wrong?' on page 18.

KEY POINTS

■ Urinary tract infections are common in women but are easily treated

■ The more serious sexually transmitted infections, such as gonorrhoea and chlamydial infection, rarely cause any symptoms in women and may not cause symptoms in a male partner either

■ Untreated genital infections may cause pelvic infections and infertility

■ A virus similar to the one that causes cold sores is responsible for genital herpes, a condition that affects 10 to 15 per cent of people

■ Visible genital warts are more of a cosmetic problem than a health hazard

■ To avoid recurrent genital infections, it is important that both partners are tested by a doctor even if only one has symptoms

■ If you have a sexually transmitted infection, it is important to get checked to make sure that you don't have other STIs

Finding out what is wrong

Where to go for help

You can obtain help from several different places where staff are qualified in the area of sexual health. They will not be shocked, embarrassed or judgemental, and will give you good advice.

General practices

Your GP's surgery is a good starting place if you have genital problems. The practice nurse may be trained in family planning and/or in dealing with genital infections. She can take swabs for infection and, together with your doctor, is often able to make a diagnosis and offer treatment before any results are available.

You may prefer to start by discussing things with the nurse. She (or he) can refer you to the doctor, or can arrange for you to see the doctor straight away if necessary.

Both of them will have details of your medical history and know about any drugs that you are taking.

This often helps them make the right diagnosis and prescribe treatment that won't interact with anything that you are already taking.

Although there are advantages to seeing someone who knows you, some people find this embarrassing with a genital problem. In this case a genitourinary medicine (GUM) clinic would be your best option; indeed, some GPs, if consulted, would suggest that you visit a GUM clinic rather than making initial investigations themselves.

Family planning clinics

The main role of a family planning clinic is to offer advice on family planning. However, staff in these clinics have been trained in a wide range of sexual health topics and are able to take swabs and offer advice. If your problem is complicated, your doctor or nurse may suggest that you should get help from your local GUM clinic.

Genitourinary medicine clinics

Most district general hospitals have a GUM clinic. If your local hospital does not have one, your GP surgery should be able to tell you where the nearest one is. Alternatively, the phone book usually has the number of your local clinic.

GUM clinics are run to diagnose and treat all types of genital problems, not only sexually transmitted ones. The doctors have undergone extensive training to specialise in this field.

The service is available to all and is confidential. Very often the diagnosis can be confirmed 'on the spot' by examining a microscope slide of secretions. Prescriptions from a GUM clinic are free of charge.

Other specialists

GPs, family planning clinics and GUM clinics all refer patients on to other specialists when the problem is outside their area of expertise. The following are other specialists who are most frequently involved in women's genital problems:

- Gynaecologists: doctors who help with menstrual problems, pelvic pain and can perform operations, if necessary

- Dermatologists: doctors who are experts in skin conditions – many run special 'vulval clinics' for specific vulval disease

- Psychosexual counsellors: who help with psychological sexual problems, such as fear of intercourse or vaginismus.

Pharmacies

Pharmacists are taught about sexual problems and can advise on medication, if appropriate, for conditions such as thrush.

Emergency contraception can be purchased from a pharmacy by women over 16 years old. Many are also able to do chlamydia tests for you and can dispense treatment for it too, if required.

Several medications suitable for genital conditions are now available over the counter in pharmacies. Examples are candida treatments, and cream for oral herpes and mild skin conditions.

What to expect?

If you have a genital problem you should, ideally, have a full genital examination, including microbiological swab tests. For specific infections, special tests are often required. For example, although swab tests for general bacterial infections may detect *Candida albicans*, they are not designed to detect chlamydial infection for which the swab must be processed in a different way.

Cervical smears are designed to detect the cell changes that increase your risk of developing cervical cancer. They can sometimes detect changes caused by thrush, warts and *Trichomonas vaginalis* (TV), but they are not the best means for testing for anything other than abnormal cervical changes.

It is therefore important to tell the doctor or nurse who is taking the swab if you have any concerns about specific symptoms or infections. They can then take the right tests to detect your infection.

Genital examination

Different doctors and nurses use different methods of examining women. The actual techniques do not matter as long as there is enough light to see your vulval skin clearly and to examine the whole of your cervix and the vaginal walls (after inserting a speculum) without causing you undue discomfort.

Routine genital examination is usually carried out with you lying on your back, legs drawn up and knees flopped open. Sometimes there are rests for your knees or heels to allow the examiner to obtain a better view.

External examination

Your vulva should be examined carefully, to look for skin discoloration or redness, discharge, ulcers and other conditions such as infected hair follicles. Most doctors would also check for enlargement or tenderness of the lymph glands (lymph nodes) in your groin.

Lymph nodes of the groin

A routine genital examination would usually check for enlargement or tenderness of lymph nodes in your groin.

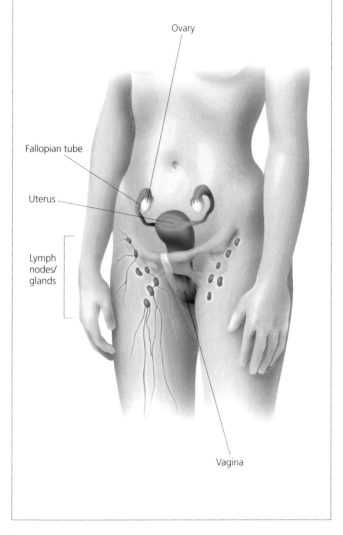

Ovary

Fallopian tube

Uterus

Lymph nodes/ glands

Vagina

Internal examination

A speculum is inserted to view your vagina and cervix, and to take swabs accurately from these areas. A speculum is usually made of metal or transparent plastic, and should ideally be warmed and lubricated so that it slips in quite painlessly (see figure on page 120). Its two halves form a shape like a duck's bill which, once inserted and gently opened, hold your vaginal walls apart so that your cervix can be seen.

Taking swabs

The doctor or nurse can look carefully at any vaginal discharge or secretions from the cervix and direct the ends of their cotton swabs to take the best specimens. Swabs are also taken from your vaginal walls to help detect vaginal infections such as candidal infection, bacterial vaginosis and trichomoniasis, and from the opening in your cervix (cervical os) to look for chlamydial infection and gonorrhoea.

The blades of the speculum are then released so that it is once more in the closed position before it is gently withdrawn. Occasionally swabs are also taken from your urethra.

Bimanual examination

After the speculum examination, or sometimes before, most doctors examine the size, shape and possible tenderness of the uterus and tubes using both their hands. This is called a bimanual examination.

It is performed by inserting two fingers into your vagina and moving your cervix to check for tenderness. At the same time the doctor puts his or her other hand on your lower abdomen to put pressure on your uterus,

Internal examination

A routine genital examination is usually carried out with you on your back with your legs open and supported. A speculum is inserted into your vagina to view and take swabs from your vagina and cervix.

View of healthy cervix

The speculum has two blades, which once opened hold your vaginal walls apart so that the cervix can be seen

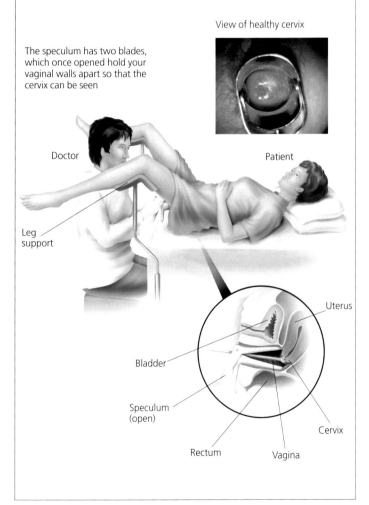

Doctor

Patient

Leg support

Uterus

Bladder

Speculum (open)

Cervix

Rectum

Vagina

so that he or she can feel your pelvic organs between his or her hands.

What if I have a small vaginal opening?

Women who have never been sexually active, and those who have not been sexually active recently, may have a tight vaginal opening, especially if they are postmenopausal. It is not always possible to examine such women and is rarely essential.

However, small 'virgin specula' are available and can be used if necessary. This tiny size can also be used if you are very anxious or very sore.

Pitfalls in examination

Examination is not always easy. The conditions in the examination room may not be ideal: the clinician may be unable to see your genitals properly, the speculum may be cold or the right swabs may not be available. The doctor or nurse may be inexperienced or nervous.

What if the doctor is male?

A male doctor, if he is not chaperoned, may be understandably reluctant to perform an intimate examination and should not normally do so except in an emergency. Similarly, you may prefer not to have a male examining you, even with a chaperone, and even if you decide to go ahead you may be too tense for him to get good specimens.

What if I am tense?

There are lots of other reasons why you may be tense. It may simply be that you are embarrassed, especially if you are not sure how private the conditions of the examination are – for example, if people keep coming

Bimanual examination

Your doctor can examine the size, shape and possible tenderness of the uterus and fallopian tubes using both hands. This is called bimanual examination and usually forms part of a routine genital examination.

A bimanual examination is performed by inserting two fingers into your vagina and moving your cervix to check for tenderness; at the same time the doctor puts his or her other hand on your lower abdomen to put pressure on your uterus, so that he or she can feel your pelvic organs between his or her hands

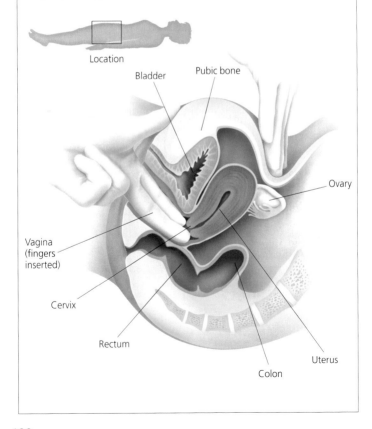

Location

Bladder

Pubic bone

Ovary

Vagina (fingers inserted)

Cervix

Rectum

Colon

Uterus

in and out of the room, or if the curtains around you are not fully drawn.

Other common reasons relate to past experiences of being touched 'down there'. For example, a previous uncomfortable examination, a bad time in childbirth or even, sadly, but quite frequently, previous sexual abuse or rape.

What will help me to relax?

It is difficult to know how to help if you feel tense about a genital examination. The doctor or nurse will try to help you by explaining how to get into the right position and make sure that you understand what is going to happen. It is important that you trust the person who is doing the examination, and that you feel calm and not hurried.

Being in the right position is also important. If you tilt your pelvis up and allow the small of your back to relax into the couch (as in the fitness exercise called pelvic tilts), your cervix is more easily visible and the examination is therefore quicker and more comfortable.

You may find that when you try to part your legs your inner thigh muscles tighten. You can try a feedback technique to control these muscles: rest your hands gently on the tendons of your inner thigh where they join your pelvis; you can then feel them as you tense and relax them. If you practise this at home first, when you are examined you will be able to tell when you are becoming tense and be better able to make a conscious effort to relax.

KEY POINTS

■ There are several different places to seek help for genital problems

■ Most hospitals have genitourinary medicine clinics that can provide specialist advice, tests and treatment

■ It is important not to delay seeking help for genital problems through fear or embarrassment; staff in GP surgeries, family planning clinics and hospital clinics are trained to deal with such feelings

Self-help for urinary and genital problems

Personal hygiene
Care with cleansing

The most important principle to remember is that your genital area is self-cleansing. Any extra cleaning that you do must be gentle and must not upset the delicate balance of micro-organisms and secretions.

If something seems wrong, you may be tempted to clean yourself more thoroughly. Washing more than once or twice a day is unnecessary and will deplete the body of its natural oils.

Washing your genitals also disrupts the waterproof film over the vulval skin, so that it becomes opaque and peels off – seeming to confirm that there was after all something abnormal to wash off. If you wash your vulva too much, it becomes more vulnerable to irritants.

Avoid irritants

The vulval skin is very sensitive to astringent liquids, such as vaginal deodorants or antiseptics, and to rubbing. Many women also find that soap, especially highly scented soap, irritates this delicate area. Plain water is best, but unperfumed soap can be used, if necessary.

Avoiding irritants can, however, be difficult. In the shower, while you may wash your genitals only with plain water, soap or shampoo used on the rest of the body can trickle down and accumulate in your vulval area. It is wise to finish a shower by cleaning your genitals with a carefully directed spray of plain water and aqueous cream.

Douching

Some women douche (using a small hose to squirt liquid into their vaginas) or use flannels or soap to clean inside their vaginas. This is not advisable because it is harmful to the normal vaginal flora and can easily cause the very infections that douching is trying to prevent.

Bladder symptoms

You can control the symptoms (but rarely eradicate the cause) of a urinary tract infection (UTI), such as passing urine too frequently and burning on passing urine, by increasing your urinary flow to flush your bladder, and by making your urine more alkaline. This makes passing urine less irritant to both the bladder wall and the urethra. 'Double micturition' and drinking cranberry juice are also worth trying (see pages 48–50).

Vulval itching or soreness

Vulval discomfort has been addressed several times in

this book (see pages 22–5, 63 and 74). What follows is general advice on soothing measures that can be used as first aid before specific treatment is started.

Avoid irritants

Once skin is inflamed, it is much more sensitive and almost anything can cause irritation. It is therefore important not to put anything, especially irritants such as astringents or antiseptic creams or washes, on the area until you know what is causing the problem.

Bathe with salt water

The best first aid for a sore or itchy vulva is bathing in salt water, in the proportions of a teaspoonful of salt (five millilitres) to half a litre of water. This is roughly the same concentration of salt as is found in blood and seawater.

Choose a washing-up bowl or similar to keep for the purpose. Fill it with salt water and sit in it for instant relief. If you have one, a bidet is ideal, but the washing-up bowl works just as well.

Your vulva can then be rinsed in the water. The results are immediate and surprisingly effective, although temporary.

Some doctors recommend adding salt to your bath. This works but it will make the rest of your skin feel dry, which you might find uncomfortable.

Keep cool and dry

It is important to keep the area cool and dry. It makes sense to allow air to circulate by wearing loose clothing, and to prevent sweat building up, by making sure that you wear clothes made of naturally absorbent material, such as cotton.

All self-help manuals recommend cotton underwear. Tight jeans are frowned on, not only because of their tightness, but because they rub.

Stockings are also recommended in place of tights, as tights are non-absorbent and prevent airflow. All these measures appear to help, although there are no scientific studies to confirm this.

If your vulva is itchy, the desire to rub or scratch may be irresistible. This is particularly true at night, so wearing cotton pants in bed can help to minimise scratching during sleep.

Over-the-counter remedies

In the most severe cases, a small oral dose of antihistamine, usually sold over the counter as a hay fever remedy, can reduce the itching and help you get a good night's sleep.

In understandable desperation, you may raid the bathroom cabinet for anything that may help your symptoms. Some things may indeed help, but they can often make the problem worse in the long run.

Creams containing steroids (such as hydrocortisone, Betnovate or Dermovate) can be very effective at temporarily damping down the inflammation. However, you should not use them unless you have specific medical advice because there is a risk that too much will be absorbed through your inflamed vulva, damaging the skin.

As inflammation is your body's response to help rid itself of infection, using any steroid cream to damp down these symptoms will tend to make fungal or viral infections worse and so is often counterproductive in the long run. This is especially important with strong steroid creams such as Betnovate and Dermovate;

General first aid measures for a sore or itchy vulva

There are a number of things that will help to relieve soreness or itching. You can use these while waiting for treatment.

- Avoid putting anything on or around the area
- Bathe the vulva in salt water (five millilitres or one teaspoon of salt to half a litre or one pint of water)
- Keep the area as cool and dry as possible
- Try to resist rubbing or scratching – especially at night

hydrocortisone is much weaker and so is less of a problem (indeed it is so weak that it is available without prescription).

If you think that you have thrush you can buy some over-the-counter remedies for it. However, if you are not sure that it is thrush, and you are planning to get tests to confirm the diagnosis, these treatments are best avoided until after the test, as prior treatment will interfere with the result.

Preventing sexually transmitted infections

The greatest risk of contracting an STI is during the first three months with a new partner. In western society, in general, most people practise 'serial monogamy' – that is, although it is uncommon to have only one sexual partner in a lifetime, most people follow the pattern of sticking to one partner for a period of time and then, after a gap, taking another. Infections can, therefore, be passed on when you change partners.

Condoms can protect against STIs but they are not infallible, nor are their users. To protect against STIs, a condom must be worn from the very start of sex play until the end of intercourse. Most infections that occur in careful condom users have been acquired from secretions during foreplay before the condom was put on.

The best way to protect yourself against STIs is to make sure that you and your new partner have a check-up at a genitourinary medicine clinic before embarking on unprotected intercourse.

KEY POINTS

- Your genital area has its own effective self-cleansing mechanism and does not need to be cleaned repeatedly or intensively

- There are various preventive and first aid measures for vulval itching or soreness

- The first three months in a new relationship carries the greatest risk of contracting an STI – condoms should always be used during this period

- Before you and your partner stop using condoms it is best for both of you to get a full check-up for STIs.

Glossary

Anaerobe: a bacterium that does not need oxygen to survive. These are found in large numbers in bacterial vaginosis (BV).

Antibody: a type of blood protein made by certain immune cells to fight an invader such as a bacterium or virus. Occasionally antibodies can, erroneously, be directed against normal parts of ourselves, as seen in autoimmune conditions.

Antibiotics: drugs that work specifically against bacteria (they do not kill viruses). The best-known example is the penicillin family of antibiotics, which kill bacteria by puncturing their cell walls. Some antibiotics attack a variety of different bacteria and are known as 'broad spectrum'. Others act only against a limited number of bacteria types and are called 'narrow spectrum'. The narrow-spectrum ones – for example, metronidazole – kill fewer types of the natural vaginal bacteria and are less likely to bring on an attack of thrush.

Asymptomatic: carrying the disease or condition but without noticing any symptoms.

Autoimmune conditions: in these conditions the body's immune system acts mistakenly against itself, usually causing inflammation and even scarring of normal tissues. Certain skin conditions are thought to be autoimmune disorders, for example, psoriasis, lichen sclerosus, Behçet's disease.

Bacteria (singular = bacterium): these are primitive life forms, less advanced than protozoa but more advanced than viruses. There are millions of different species (types). In the genital area, they cause infections such as urinary tract infections (UTIs), bacterial vaginosis and infected hair follicles. They can be killed by antibiotics.

Bacterial vaginosis (BV): a condition of bacterial imbalance in the vagina often causing a fishy smelling discharge.

Behçet's disease: a rare condition where there may be ulcers on the genitals and in the mouth. There are often other problems such as inflamed veins.

Biopsy: a small sample of tissue. This is removed after numbing the area with an anaesthetic. The sample is then sent for examination under the microscope to diagnose what is wrong.

Cervical canal: the hole in the cervix leading to the internal cavity of the uterus (womb).

Cervix (Latin = neck): neck of the womb (uterus). Acts like a muscular band at the base of the uterus, keeping the developing fetus (baby) inside.

Colonisation: settlement of micro-organisms on or in the body, where they live without causing any harm.

Columnar epithelium: a particular type of skin that lines some hollow parts of the body such as the uterus. It spreads slightly over the surface of the cervix and joins the skin of the vagina (squamous epithelium) at the squamocolumnar junction.

Crohn's disease: a rare disorder of the gut that may cause pain, bleeding and diarrhoea. People are often also generally unwell and sometimes develop painful sores and swellings around their anus and on their genitals.

Cystitis: a term often used to describe a bacterial urinary tract infection. The Greek name for a bladder is cystis and this has been used for the bladder in medical terminology – hence cystitis strictly speaking means inflammation of the bladder alone. Inflammation can result from other things such as chemotherapy drugs, so cystitis does not always mean that infection is present.

Dysuria: pain on passing urine, usually felt as urine comes out of the bladder, as a result of irritation of the urethra.

Dyspareunia: pain on sexual intercourse. It can be divided into pain on the outside (superficial dyspareunia) and pain felt deep in the pelvis (deep dyspareunia).

Ectopy: area of columnar epithelium on the vaginal part of the cervix, which produces mucus secretions. It is usually found at times in reproductive life when oestrogen levels are highest, for example, pregnancy.

Eczema: the word just means inflamed skin. However, it is usually used to mean inflamed skin caused by an allergy or with no obvious cause. This type of eczema is often found on more than one part of the body.

Endometriosis: in this condition, small patches of the lining material of the uterus are found outside their normal place. Symptoms include painful periods (where pain usually starts before the onset of bleeding), dyspareunia and, when severe, infertility.

Epithelium (Latin = skin): surface layers of the skin or any membranous lining.

False negative: a negative test result that is inaccurate, and has occurred even though the condition tested for is present.

False positive: a positive result that has occurred even though the condition tested for is absent.

Fibroids: knots of muscle in the uterus or sticking out from its walls. There are often no symptoms, although fibroids can cause heavy, painful periods and infertility. Fibroids are common, especially in older women.

Flora: the collection of microbes in the vagina is known by the same term as that used for a collection of plants. The 'normal flora' is the highly complex but balanced constituents of a normal vagina.

Genitourinary medicine (GUM): the name for the medical specialty dealing in genital problems and sexually transmitted infections. GUM clinics are found in most large hospitals and offer expert advice and confidential tests for all STIs.

Herpes simplex virus (HSV): the name for the virus that causes genital herpes and cold sores.

Human papilloma virus (HPV): the group name for viruses that cause a variety of warts in humans. Certain members of this group are confined to the genitals – especially types 6, 11, 16, 18 and 32.

Hyfrecation: a treatment for warts. After the area has been numbed with an anaesthetic, warts are gently scraped off the normal skin using a tiny red-hot wire.

Incubation: the process in which, for example, a culture of bacteria is kept in the ideal conditions to allow them to grow and be identified.

Incubation period: the time between catching an infection and symptoms developing.

Inflammation: the normal reaction of the body to an infection or to damage. There is redness and swelling and, if it is very severe, the area may ooze or weep clear fluid, or even pus and blood. It can also occur in autoimmune diseases where the body's own antibodies react against its own tissues. Inflammation, although usually present with infection, can also occur when there is no infection.

Introitus: external visible opening of the vagina.

Irritable bowel syndrome: this is a condition in which the walls of the bowel become sensitive and tend to go into painful spasms, or just become generally tender. It is a very common cause of pelvic pain in young women. It should always be considered when the pain is long lasting, especially if there are also bowel symptoms such as diarrhoea or constipation.

Labia (Latin for lips; singular = labium): the lips of the vulva. There are two pairs: the outer, usually larger ones – the labia majora – and the inner, usually smaller, ones – the labia minora.

Lichen simplex: a skin condition where the skin becomes thickened and itchy – often as a result of rubbing.

Lymph nodes (glands): part of the body's immune system. Lymph nodes in the groin can sometimes be felt on the front of the panty line and, if there is infection on the vulva, they may swell and become painful to touch.

Menopause: commonly known as the 'change of life'. The time when oestrogen hormone levels drop and menstruation stops. The average age when this occurs for women in the UK is 51 years.

Micro-organisms: another name for microbes. Those dealt with here are (starting with the most primitive): viruses such as herpes; bacteria such as those that cause BV or urine infections; yeasts such as *Candida albicans* (thrush); and protozoa such as *Trichomonas vaginalis*.

Microscopy: the use of a microscope to look at micro-organisms such as bacteria. Microscopy of vaginal secretions is done to look for thrush, BV or gonorrhoea.

Molluscum contagiosum (Latin = contagious snails!): a virus infection that causes small, round, shiny spots that resemble small pearl-like snails. They can form on any part of the body but often appear on the genitals in adults. They can be caught from a sexual partner, but they are also commonly spread by any direct body contact, especially in children. They can be confused with warts.

Mycelium (plural = mycelia): microscopic strands of fungal growth as seen in the vagina when there is active candidal infection.

Oestrogen: a female hormone that increases at puberty and in pregnancy and decreases after the menopause. It is a constituent of the combined oral contraceptive pill.

Ovulation: midway in the menstrual cycle, a follicle (like a tiny cyst) in the ovary ruptures to release an egg (ovum) ready for fertilisation. Sometimes this ruptured follicle can bleed and cause 'midcycle pain'.

Papilloma (Greek = a swelling): warty growth. The word can be used to describe wart-like growths anywhere in the body, but most often it is used in connection with the bladder. Bladder papillomas can develop into cancer and need to be removed.

Pelvic inflammatory disease (PID): infection of the uterus and fallopian tubes, usually caused by chlamydial infection or gonorrhoea, can lead to infertility.

Predisposing factors: these factors are things that, if present, make something else more likely to happen; in other words they are risk factors. For example, antibiotic treatment will predispose to (make more likely) an attack of thrush.

Prodrome: the symptoms that come before a full-blown attack of a disease. In the prodrome of herpes, there is usually a combination of some of the following: malaise, pains and tingling down the back, aching in the thighs and tingling at the site where the herpes sore is going to develop.

Progesterone: a female hormone that increases at puberty and in pregnancy and decreases after the menopause. Progesterone is contained in all contraceptive pills including the mini-pill and in the menopause hormone replacement treatment (HRT). It is also the active ingredient in contraceptive injections, implants and the progesterone-containing intrauterine device (coil), Mirena.

Protozoa (Latin, singular = protozoan): micro-organisms that consist of one cell, and are one level more advanced than bacteria. Examples are *Trichomonas* and *Amoeba*.

Pyelonephritis: a kidney infection, which has usually spread from an infected bladder.

Recurrences: repeated attacks of a condition.

Secretion: fluid that oozes, usually in very small quantities, from body tissues. The source of the fluid is either secretory glands, the function of which is to produce fluid, or inflamed tissues that are reacting to some irritant.

Speculum (Latin = mirror): an instrument used to look inside the vagina.

Squamocolumnar junction: the place where squamous and columnar epithelia meet on the cervix. The actual level of the join varies through life and is the area where, in those at risk, cervical cancer can develop.

Squamous epithelium: the type of skin that lines the vagina and extends up as far as the lower part of the cervix.

Swabs: swabs are sterile cotton buds that are used to soak up samples of secretions so that they can be sent to the lab for testing. Most people will have experienced having a throat swab taken to detect bacteria when they have a sore throat. A similar process is carried out using swabs inserted into the vagina or urethra to test for the presence of genital infections.

Symptom: an indication that something is wrong with your body or the way you are feeling. A symptom is something you notice about yourself, for example, a pain or a lump.

Trichomonas vaginalis (TV): a protozoan that causes an infection of the vagina, resulting in soreness and discharge.

Ureter: a tube that carries urine from each kidney to the bladder, where it is then stored until it is passed out through the urethra. There are two ureters (right and left) in the body.

Urethra: the tube down which urine flows from the bladder to the outside. It opens on to the vulva in women.

Urinary tract infection (UTI): infection of part or all of the urinary tract, almost always caused by bacteria. The urinary tract includes the kidneys, ureters, bladder and urethra. Usually, infection is confined to the bladder and urethra – the term is sometimes used interchangeably with 'cystitis'.

Vaginismus: spasm of the thigh and pelvic muscles, which prevents penetration of the vagina.

Viruses: infectious organisms that are among the most primitive life forms on earth. On the genitals, they cause conditions such as herpes and genital warts. There is no effective treatment for most viruses (aciclovir for herpes is a rare exception); they are not killed by antibiotics.

Vulva: the external, visible area of skin that consists of the clitoris, the opening of the urethra, the two pairs of lips (labia minora and labia majora) and the opening of the vagina (introitus).

Vulvodynia (Greek = painful vulva): a poorly understood condition, the main symptom of which is a burning pain of the vulva. There is nothing to see and tests don't show any cause. It usually gets better over time.

Useful addresses

Where can I find out more?

We have included the following organisations because, on preliminary investigation, they may be of use to the reader. However, we do not have first-hand experience of each organisation and so cannot guarantee the organisation's integrity. The reader must therefore exercise his or her own discretion and judgement when making further enquiries.

Benefits Enquiry Line

Tel: 0800 882200
Minicom: 0800 243355
Website: www.dwp.gov.uk
N. Ireland: 0800 220674
Minicom: 0800 243789

Government agency giving information and advice on sickness and disability for people with disabilities and their carers.

Brook

Studio 421, Highgate Studios
53–79 Highgate Road
London NW5 1TL
Tel: 020 7284 6040
Fax: 020 7284 6050
Email: admin@brookcentres.org.uk
Helpline: 0800 018 5023 (9am–5pm)
Website: www.brook.org.uk

Offers free, confidential helpline to young people up to 25 years on contraception, sexual health and personal relationships. Can refer to local centres. Recorded information also available on 020 7950 7700.

Citizens Advice Bureaux

Myddelton House, 115–123 Pentonville Road
London N1 9LZ
Tel: 020 7833 2181 (admin only)
Website: www.adviceguide.org.uk

HQ of national charity offering a wide variety of practical, financial and legal advice. Network of local charities throughout the UK listed in phone books and in *Yellow Pages* under 'C'.

Endometriosis SHE Trust (UK)

14 Moorland Way
Lincoln LN6 7JW
Tel: 08707 743665
Email: shetrust@shetrust.org.uk
Website: www.shetrust.org.uk

Offers support to women with endometriosis and information about medical, surgical, complementary and nutritional treatments. Publishes leaflets and newsletters for members.

Herpes Viruses Association

41 North Road
London N7 9DP
Tel: 020 7607 9661
Fax: 020 7700 1171
Helpline: 0845 123 2305
Email: info@herpes.org.uk
Website: www.herpes.org.uk

Offers information and support to people with herpes viruses. Organises seminars, social events and can refer to local self-help contacts. Supplies details of self-help and medical treatment for shingles and post-herpetic neuralgia. An SAE requested.

The Cystitis and Overactive Bladder Foundation

76 High Street
Stony Stratford, Bucks MK11 1AH
Tel: 01908 569169
Fax: 01908 565665
Email: info@cobfoundation.org
Website: www.cobfoundation.org

Offers videos and information for health professionals and people with interstitial cystitis and their families and friends. Can refer to local support groups and individuals.

National Institute for Health and Clinical Excellence

MidCity Place, 71 High Holborn
London WC1V 6NA
Tel: 020 7067 5800
Fax: 020 7067 5801
Email: nice@nice.org.uk
Website: www.nice.org.uk

Provides national guidance on the promotion of good health and the prevention and treatment of ill-health. Patient information leaflets are available for each piece of guidance issued.

NHS Direct

Tel: 0845 4647 (24 hours, 365 days a year)
Website: www.nhsdirect.nhs.uk
NHS Scotland: 0800 224488
Textphone: 0845 606 4647

Offers confidential health-care advice, information and referral service. Good first port of call for any health advice.

NHS Smoking Helpline

Tel: 0800 169 0169 (7am-–11pm, 365 days a year)
Website: www.givingupsmoking.co.uk
Pregnancy smoking helpline: 0800 169 9169
(12noon–9pm, 365 days a year)
N. Ireland: 0800 858585 (12noon–10pm, 365 days a year)
Scotland: 0800 848484 (12noon–12midnight, 365 days a year)
Wales: 0800 085 2219

Have advice, help and encouragement on giving up smoking. Specialist advisers available to offer on-going support to those who genuinely are trying to give up smoking. Can refer to local branches.

Prodigy Website
Sowerby Centre for Health Informatics at Newcastle (SCHIN), Bede House
All Saints Business Centre
Newcastle upon Tyne NE1 2ES
Tel: 0191 243 6100
Fax: 0191 243 6101
Email: prodigy-enquiries@schin.co.uk
Website: www.prodigy.nhs.uk

A website mainly for GPs giving information for patients listed by disease plus named self-help organisations.

Quit (Smoking Quitlines)
211 Old Street
London EC1V 9NR
Helpline: 0800 00 22 00 (9am–9pm, 365 days a year)
Tel: 020 7251 1551
Fax: 020 7251 1661
Email: info@quit.org.uk
Website: www.quit.org.uk

Offers individual advice on giving up smoking in English and Asian languages. Talks to schools on smoking and can refer to local support groups. Runs training courses for professionals.

Women's Health Concern Ltd

Whitehall House, 41 Whitehall
London SW1A 2BY
Tel: 020 7451 1377
Fax: 020 7925 1505
Help line: 0845 123 2319 (Mon–Fri 9am–5pm)
Email: info@womens-health-concern.org
Website: www.womens-health-concern.org
Website for menopausal queries:
www.menopausematters.co.uk

Offers information, advice and counselling to women
with gynaecological and hormonal problems. Send an
SAE for current list of publications.

Useful link

www.womenshealthlondon.org.uk

Information leaflets about gynaecological and sexual
health issues can be downloaded.

The internet as a further source of information

After reading this book, you may feel that you would
like further information on the subject. The internet is
of course an excellent place to look and there are
many websites with useful information about medical
disorders, related charities and support groups.

For those who do not have a computer at home
some bars and cafes offer facilities for accessing the
internet. These are listed in the *Yellow Pages* under
'Internet Bars and Cafes' and 'Internet Providers'. Your
local library offers a similar facility and has staff to help
you find the information that you need.

It should always be remembered, however, that the internet is unregulated and anyone is free to set up a website and add information to it. Many websites offer impartial advice and information that has been compiled and checked by qualified medical professionals. Some, on the other hand, are run by commercial organisations with the purpose of promoting their own products. Others still are run by pressure groups, some of which will provide carefully assessed and accurate information whereas others may be suggesting medications or treatments that are not supported by the medical and scientific community.

Unless you know the address of the website you want to visit – for example, www.familydoctor.co.uk – you may find the following guidelines useful when searching the internet for information.

Search engines and other searchable sites

Google (www.google.co.uk) is the most popular search engine used in the UK, followed by Yahoo! (http://uk.yahoo.com) and MSN (www.msn.co.uk). Also popular are the search engines provided by Internet Service Providers such as Tiscali and other sites such as the BBC site (www.bbc.co.uk).

In addition to the search engines that index the whole web, there are also medical sites with search facilities, which act almost like mini-search engines, but cover only medical topics or even a particular area of medicine. Again, it is wise to look at who is responsible for compiling the information offered to ensure that it is impartial and medically accurate. The NHS Direct site (www.nhsdirect.nhs.uk) is an example of a searchable medical site.

Links to many British medical charities can be found at the websites for the Association of Medical Research Charities (www.amrc.org.uk) and Charity Choice (www.charitychoice.co.uk).

Search phrases

Be specific when entering a search phrase. Searching for information on 'cancer' will return results for many different types of cancer as well as on cancer in general. You may even find sites offering astrological information. More useful results will be returned by using search phrases such as 'lung cancer' and 'treatments for lung cancer'. Both Google and Yahoo! offer an advanced search option that includes the ability to search for the exact phrase, enclosing the search phrase in quotes, that is, 'treatments for lung cancer' will have the same effect. Limiting a search to an exact phrase reduces the number of results returned but it is best to refine a search to an exact match only if you are not getting useful results with a normal search. Adding 'UK' to your search term will bring up mainly British sites, so a good phrase might be 'lung cancer' UK (don't include UK within the quotes).

Always remember the internet is international and unregulated. It holds a wealth of valuable information but individual sites may be biased, out of date or just plain wrong. Family Doctor Publications accepts no responsibility for the content of links published in this series.

Index

Your pages

We have included the following pages because they may help you manage your illness or condition and its treatment.

Before an appointment with a health professional, it can be useful to write down a short list of questions of things that you do not understand, so that you can make sure that you do not forget anything.

Some of the sections may not be relevant to your circumstances.

We are always pleased to receive constructive criticism or suggestions about how to improve the books. You can contact us at:

Email: familydoctor@btinternet.com
Letter: Family Doctor Publications
         PO Box 4664
         Poole
         BH15 1NN

Thank you

Health-care contact details

Name:

Job title:

Place of work:

Tel:

Name:

Job title:

Place of work:

Tel:

Name:

Job title:

Place of work:

Tel:

Name:

Job title:

Place of work:

Tel:

Significant past health events – illnesses/ operations/investigations/treatments

Event	Month	Year	Age (at time)

Appointments for health care

Name:

Place:

Date:

Time:

Tel:

Name:

Place:

Date:

Time:

Tel:

Name:

Place:

Date:

Time:

Tel:

Name:

Place:

Date:

Time:

Tel:

Appointments for health care

Name:

Place:

Date:

Time:

Tel:

Name:

Place:

Date:

Time:

Tel:

Name:

Place:

Date:

Time:

Tel:

Name:

Place:

Date:

Time:

Tel:

Current medication(s) prescribed by your doctor

Medicine name:

Purpose:

Frequency & dose:

Start date:

End date:

Medicine name:

Purpose:

Frequency & dose:

Start date:

End date:

Medicine name:

Purpose:

Frequency & dose:

Start date:

End date:

Medicine name:

Purpose:

Frequency & dose:

Start date:

End date:

Other medicines/supplements you are taking, not prescribed by your doctor

Medicine/treatment:

Purpose:

Frequency & dose:

Start date:

End date:

Medicine/treatment:

Purpose:

Frequency & dose:

Start date:

End date:

Medicine/treatment:

Purpose:

Frequency & dose:

Start date:

End date:

Medicine/treatment:

Purpose:

Frequency & dose:

Start date:

End date:

Questions to ask at appointments
(Note: do bear in mind that doctors work under great time pressure, so long lists may not be helpful for either of you)

Questions to ask at appointments
(Note: do bear in mind that doctors work under great time pressure, so long lists may not be helpful for either of you)

Notes